Menopause

Menopause

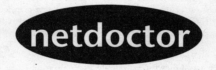

Series Editor
Dr Dan Rutherford
www.netdoctor.co.uk

Hodder & Stoughton
LONDON SYDNEY AUCKLAND

Copyright © 2003 by NetDoctor.co.uk
Illustrations copyright © 2003 by Amanda Williams

First published in Great Britain in 2003

The right of NetDoctor.co.uk to be identified as the Author
of the Work has been asserted by them in accordance
with the Copyright, Designs and Patents Act 1988.

10 9 8 7 6 5 4 3 2

British Library Cataloguing in Publication Data
A record for this book is available from the British Library

ISBN 0 340 86140 1

Typeset in Garamond by Avon DataSet Ltd,
Bidford-on-Avon, Warwickshire

Printed and bound in Great Britain by
Bookmarque Ltd., Croydon, Surrey

The paper and board used in this paperback are natural recyclable
products made from wood grown in sustainable forests.
The manufacturing processes conform to the environmental
regulations of the country of origin.

Hodder & Stoughton
A Division of Hodder Headline Ltd
338 Euston Road
London NW1 3BH
www.madaboutbooks.com

Contents

Foreword

In the UK and many other western countries one of the most dramatic occurrences of the 20th century was the marked increase in life expectancy. A British woman can now anticipate living, on average, more than 80 years. In contrast, the average age of menopause is around 50 years and has remained so since it was first documented centuries ago. Therefore much of a woman's life will be lived after the menopause. Women's expectations of older age are now high and most want to do all they can to remain active and healthy, leading an enjoyable life and playing a useful role in society.

The last 10–20 years have seen a huge surge of interest in the menopause, both from the medical perspective and from the needs of the individual woman. Problems associated with the menopause are now much more openly discussed. Hormone replacement therapy (HRT) has become a household name and most women will value the opportunity to discuss, with a healthcare professional, the possibility of taking HRT. It will definitely control the unpleasant hot flushes and sweats associated with the menopause and improve the quality of a woman's life at this stage. However, whether HRT should be used for the prevention of conditions such as heart disease and stroke, osteoporosis or Alzheimer's disease has become much more controversial. Only more medical research over the next few decades can answer these questions. We know also that HRT can cause side effects and for some women the disadvantages of HRT outweigh the advantages. Women as a result have been seeking alternatives to HRT in the form of 'natural' herbal cures but should be aware that many of these 'natural' remedies have their own side effects and are of no proven benefit.

For the menopausal woman stopping smoking, taking more exercise and having a healthy diet are of definite value to her long-term health. These are all actions that are part of 'menopause treatment' too.

This book gives an exceptionally balanced view of the menopause and I recommend it wholeheartedly to all women in the UK approaching their menopausal years. We are constantly bombarded with sensation-alised newspaper headlines and biased magazine articles on the meno-pause and straightforward, highly informative books like this are to be truly welcomed.

Dr Ailsa E. Gebbie MB, ChB, MRCOG, MFFP
Consultant Gynaecologist, Lothian Primary Care NHS Trust, Edinburgh
and Honorary Senior Lecturer, Department of Clinical Sciences and
Community Health, University of Edinburgh

Acknowledgements

I am very pleased indeed to acknowledge the invaluable help I've been given in the preparation of this book by Dr Ailsa Gebbie of the Family Planning and Well Woman Services in Edinburgh. As a leading menopause expert for over 15 years she was well placed to help advise on the facts, and did so with great care and attention despite her busy schedule.

Equally busy but just as cheerful, enthusiastic and helpful an adviser has been Dr Hilary McPherson MB, ChB, MRCOG, DCH, MBA (Healthcare), Consultant Gynaecologist at the Simpson Centre for Reproductive Health in the Royal Infirmary of Edinburgh. I thank Ailsa and Hilary for ensuring that this book is not only accurate but that it is written in a way that is sympathetic to a woman's viewpoint.

I thank Dr John Dean for his original writings on the NetDoctor website that formed the basis of the chapter on the 'male menopause'.

As always, I am indebted to the editorial team at Hodder & Stoughton who get less credit than they deserve. Judith and Julie in particular – thanks again.

If any errors have crept in to this book despite our best efforts, then please let me know. We also welcome suggestions for improvements to this or any of the other books in the series. I can be contacted at d.rutherford@netdoctor.co.uk

Dr Dan Rutherford
Medical Director
www.netdoctor.co.uk

Chapter 1

What Is the Menopause?

Introduction

The basic definition of the menopause is that time in a woman's life when she has stopped menstruating. In Western societies this usually occurs within the age range of 45 to 55, the average being about 51 years. As with most human characteristics there is a wide range of 'normal'. Some women experience the menopause in their 30s whereas others continue menstruating into their 60s.

Menstruation occurs when the egg released by one of the two ovaries fails in that menstrual cycle to be fertilised. The ensuing hormone changes cause the shedding of the lining of the uterus (womb), in order for the process to repeat itself and prepare the uterus to receive a fertilised egg in the next cycle. The menopause is therefore the outward sign that ovarian function has declined and that the woman is past her reproductive years.

Occasionally it is necessary to surgically remove both functioning ovaries, and when this happens a woman is propelled into the menopause right away. However, the natural process of ovarian 'failure' is generally a gradual process that can take as many as five years to finally end with the complete absence of menstruation. During this period of time a woman can experience a range of symptoms that are caused by the decline of the hormone output of the ovaries. This phase of life leading up to the menopause is often called the 'climacteric', or the 'peri-menopause'.

The familiar symptoms of the menopause, such as flushes and sweats, are the result of the drop in hormone production by the ovaries and they can occur during the climacteric phase, even when the menstrual cycle itself still occurs regularly. As the climacteric progresses, however, there is also a gradual lengthening of the time between periods, or an irregular pattern of menstrual bleeding in which long and short cycles occur randomly. Generally the amount of blood lost in each period drops as the true menopause is approached, before it finally falls to zero.

At the menopause the ovaries permanently cease to produce eggs. The ways in which the ovaries are controlled to develop and release the eggs during a woman's reproductive years are now quite well understood and include a complex interplay of hormones that also involves the brain and the bloodstream. It is useful to know the essentials of this system in order to fully understand the menopause and so this is covered in the next chapter.

Before getting to the scientific details it is, however, important to consider the menopause in a wider context.

Medical condition or natural process?

Every woman who lives long enough will experience the menopause. It is therefore a natural part of aging. Why then is there so much medical interest in it? Many people are of the opinion that the menopause has become 'over-medicalised' and has almost attracted the status of a disease rather than a normal phase of a woman's life. There is much to support this view. Among the most obvious points of criticism are the recent shifts in medical opinion concerning the 'benefits' of treatment of the menopause, particularly with respect to hormone replacement therapy (HRT). Putting it mildly, it is fair to say that some of the previously assumed benefits of HRT do not look now to be as convincing as they were thought to be a few years ago. Putting it more strongly, others might say that the results of several recent major trials of HRT have put the whole matter into confusion and disarray. We'll attempt to make sense of this later.

Some perhaps overly cynical critics believe that the considerable pharmaceutical company interest that results from considering the menopause to be a medical condition (and for which prescription drugs can therefore be manufactured and dispensed) is partly respon-sible for our present position. Equally though, it is important not to lose sight of the fact that getting older brings its consequences, which for a woman include those that result from ovarian decline. Many women undoubtedly gain benefit from treatment for this.

Although only a proportion of women may need or will potentially benefit from menopause treatment, every woman needs to know enough about the menopause to make an informed decision about what action, if any, she needs to take. The main aim of this book is to help provide that level of understanding.

Benefits of the menopause

One of the consequences of the 'medical' approach is that the menopause assumes the qualities of a disease, with an associated list of symptoms. There's a general principle that diseases are bad, and by implication so too must be the menopause. For many women this is far from true.

Freedom from the routine of menstrual bleeding, from the need to worry about contraception or from having to deal with pre-menstrual mood swings and bloating are seen by most as a benefit rather than a disadvantage.

Historically the menopause has coincided with the time in a woman's life when her children are leaving home, thus leading to the so-called 'empty nest syndrome' in which there is the double whammy of the loss of reproductive status combined with the 'loss' of the children. Such a scenario is, however, recognised by only a minority of women in our modern society; many are more likely to value the increased freedom that a quieter household brings with it.

Well-being

Well-being is harder to define than disease. It is relatively easy to quote the symptoms known to be associated with the menopause but harder to list what constitutes well-being when there are so many other important issues in a woman's life at this time.

If a woman sees herself as attractive, is engaged in a rewarding job or has a stable and supportive relationship with her partner she is likely to experience fewer menopause-related problems than a woman with low self-esteem, who is unhappy with her appearance, who has an unsatisfactory relationship or who has an unstable or unsupportive social network. Being employed and valued are protective factors against the psychological ill effects of the menopause. The menopause is clearly not just about ovaries and hormones; it's also about life in general. Keeping this in mind is a good idea when considering what might be causing the problems a woman experiences around the menopause. An overly superficial belief (on the part of the doctor as well as the patient) that hormone deficiency is the problem and replacement the answer will probably result in disappointment all round when such treatment fails to deliver the expected results.

Am I menopausal?

This is a common and very reasonable question. As the definition of the menopause is the natural cessation of periods then it is superficially easy to answer. An arbitrary length of time (6 to 12 months depending on who you ask) is chosen as the marker, and if a period hasn't come in this length of time then one assumes they're not going to. However, that's not really what the question is usually about. What most women mean is 'are the problems I'm presently experiencing due to the menopause?'. Women also commonly want to know if there is a 'test' for the menopause, i.e. something objective that the doctor can do that categorically states one way or the other if the menopause is present, and if so whether it is problematic. Unfortunately it's not that easy to be sure.

First there is the climacteric, itself sometimes years long, in which periods still happen and during which the symptoms of the menopause start to appear. So going on the absence of periods alone is not a lot of help during this phase. Second is the woman who hasn't had periods for the 'required' number of months but who hasn't had many problem symptoms either – is she menopausal? Third is the woman who is some years older than when she last had a period – technically she is post-menopausal, but how does she know if she needs to do anything about it?

It would be a boon if we had tests that could tell which women were suffering problems from the menopause or climacteric, or would pick out those who would benefit from treatment. Additionally it would be very helpful if we had indicators that showed how long menopause treatment should last. We don't have any such tests. The evidence pointing towards or away from the menopause being the source of certain symptoms or other difficulties has to be gathered bit by bit. It is the overall picture that counts, and even then it might not be certain that the menopause is the issue. Using a trial of treatment with hormone replacement therapy (HRT, see later) can help a bit further – those women who benefit from the treatment might be said to have had the case confirmed that it was 'the hormones' that were causing the problems in the first place, but this is not a reliable way of detecting everyone who should receive HRT.

If this seems like a slightly confusing picture, it is true that it is, at least to some extent! However, it is possible to make sense of it and this will become clearer during the course of the book. The symptoms of the menopause is the logical place to start.

The symptoms of the menopause

In an attempt to add some structure to assessing a woman's symptoms and determining whether they are due to the menopause a small number of 'rating scales' have been developed that list the main symptoms, and against which one can mark the degree to which they are experienced by an individual. Totting up the score gives some indication of how much trouble the menopause may be causing. The previous few paragraphs have touched on the potential pitfalls of such an approach. Human beings are complicated and don't easily reduce down to numbers on a tick chart, but symptoms scores are useful if they are taken as a guide and not as gospel.

The menopause rating scale (MRS) is one such questionnaire-based scoring system focussing on 11 symptom items. In the full questionnaire each symptom is given a mark depending on the degree of severity from 0 (no symptom) to 3 (severe symptoms):

Table 1: Overview of the 'menopause rating scale' items

1 Hot flushes, episodes of sweating
2 'Heart' symptoms (unusual awareness of the heartbeat, heart skipping a beat or racing)
3 Sleep problems (difficulty falling asleep or sleeping through the night, waking early)

4　Depressive symptoms (feeling down, tearful, lacking motivation, mood swings)

5　Irritability (nervousness, inner tension, feeling aggressive)

6　Anxiety (inner restlessness, feeling panicky)

7　Physical and mental exhaustion (general decrease in performance, impaired memory, decrease in concentration, forgetfulness)

8　Sexual problems (change in sexual desire, in amount of sexual activity and degree of satisfaction)

9　Bladder problems (difficulty in passing urine, increased need to pass urine, incontinence)

10　Dryness of vagina (sensation of dryness or burning, difficulty with sexual intercourse)

11　Joint and muscle discomfort

Taken individually each of these symptoms of course has other possible explanations. Heart racing could be due to anaemia (low blood count), anxiety or an over-active thyroid gland for example. Bladder frequency could be due to cystitis (bladder infection) or diabetes among other causes. Sleep disturbance could be secondary to depression and so on. A doctor naturally has to assess these symptoms and the likelihood of alternative causes – self-diagnosis is not recommended. However, the more of these symptoms that are present, and the greater their severity, the higher the chance that it is the menopause that has brought them together in a particular woman.

This is not a complete list of all possible symptoms that can be associated with the menopause, but it forms a useful checklist of the most characteristic ones. The commonest symptoms are hot flushes and night sweats, which in a minority of women are severe. Less common are psychological symptoms such as impaired memory and mood disturbance, general symptoms such as fatigue, bladder or vaginal symptoms and a lack of sexual interest. Exactly how much less common is, however, more difficult to say. Flushes and sweats may be intolerable enough to take a woman to her doctor in the search for advice or treatment, but matters such as a lack of libido or a dry vagina during intercourse get mentioned less often, even if they are present as a problem. There is still a reluctance to discuss sexual issues in our society. A doctor sufficiently in tune with the potential problems of the menopause will ask relevant questions directly about such matters, and the majority of women welcome the opportunity to discuss them.

Menopause and health checks

Going to the doctor to talk about the menopause is also an opportunity for a woman to consider her health in a wider context. In middle age the effects of other health-related factors such as a high fat diet, excess body weight, smoking, raised blood pressure and cholesterol and a sedentary lifestyle begin to have more obvious impacts. The greater the number of these so-called 'risk factors' for developing heart and blood vessel diseases that are present in an individual the greater the degree of risk. Conversely, relatively small changes for the better in these risk factors can have substantial health benefits. The chance can and should therefore be taken to ensure that these important health issues are checked and that appropriate advice is made available when needed. This is all the more important at the menopause because oestrogen, one of the main hormones produced by the active ovaries, has a protective effect upon the heart and blood vessels (cardiovascular system) of the pre-menopausal woman. Following the menopause this protective effect is lost and so one sees an increase in cardiovascular disease in menopausal women. We'll come later to more discussion of this issue.

Screening

Routine cervical screening (smear test) is offered to women in the UK between the ages of 20 and 60 and breast screening (mammogram) between 50 and 64. Mammography is not routinely offered to younger women for several reasons, including the fact that most women under 50 are pre-menopausal. The breast tissue before the menopause is denser and harder to interpret for abnormalities by mammogram. This is also a factor to be considered in hormone replacement, which also causes increased breast tissue density and increases the likelihood of breast cancer developing (see chapter 6 for more details). Breast screening can be extended to later ages at the woman's request and there are plans to extend routine breast screening in the UK to the age of 70 by 2004.

These are familiar tests and most women take advantage of them. The proportion of women who have other health screening tests done is, however, smaller. Women are less likely than men to have had a check of their cholesterol level, despite the fact that raised cholesterol is just as bad for women after the menopause as it is for men at any time.

More information on the broader aspects of healthy living, including those other tests that are worth having, are in the companion book in this series, entitled *How to Stay Healthy*.

Key Points

- The menopause is the natural cessation of menstrual periods, which on average occurs at the age of 51 in Western women.
- The menopause is caused by the decline in function of the ovaries, which can take from several months to several years to occur.
- The phase around the time of the completed menopause is called the climacteric, or peri-menopause.
- Only a proportion of women may need or will potentially benefit from menopause treatment.
- Hot flushes and sweats are the commonest of the many symptoms that can be associated with the menopause.
- Other important general health issues should be considered alongside the menopause.

Chapter 2

Hormones and the Body

Hormones in general

Hormones are substances produced in one part of the body that have effects on tissues elsewhere in the body. They reach their 'target' tissues via the bloodstream. There are many known hormones, with a wide range of important effects. For example, insulin produced by the pancreas gland inside the abdomen is the main hormone responsible for controlling the level of glucose (sugar) in the blood. Thyroid hormone produced by the thyroid gland in the neck controls the body's general rate of metabolism. Of particular interest in relation to the menopause are the sex hormones, which technically are types of steroid.

'Steroid' is the general name for a group of similar compounds that have profound effects on the body. The main female sex hormones are oestrogen and progesterone and the main male sex hormone is testosterone. All of the steroid molecules have a structure that is chemically similar to cholesterol, and most are synthesised in the body from cholesterol as the starting point, thus emphasising one of the important roles of this essential substance – it does a lot more than fur up our arteries.

The sex hormones

These are thus described because of their importance in directing the sexual development of the growing embryo at the start of life and for their further effects in driving sexual maturity at puberty. Oestrogen and progesterone are produced by the ovaries in females and testosterone by the testes in males, although not exclusively. Small amounts of oestrogen and progesterone are produced normally by males in the testes and small amounts of testosterone by women in the ovaries. In both sexes small steroid-producing glands above the kidneys (the adrenal glands) produce a wider range of other steroids too. There is, however, a marked difference in sensitivity to the sex hormones between the sexes. Women are very sensitive to small increases in testosterone for example, which if present can cause male features to appear, such as hair growth on the chin. Despite the many differences in the actions of these hormones their chemical structures are remarkably similar.

Sex hormone control

The sex hormone system in both sexes has a hierarchy of three levels:

1 The top level is an area deep in the middle part of the brain, called the hypothalamus.
2 Underneath the hypothalamus and connected to it by a short stalk of nerve fibres and blood vessels is the pituitary gland. About the

size of a small grape, its importance far outweighs its dimensions. Among the many hormones produced by the pituitary gland are follicle-stimulating hormone (FSH) and luteinising hormone (LH). FSH and LH are released into the bloodstream via the network of blood vessels that go through the pituitary gland and in this way they reach their targets – the gonads (ovaries and testes).

3 The ovaries and testes manufacture the bulk of the relevant sex hormones and release them into the bloodstream.

LH and FSH in men control the output of testosterone and regulate the development of sperm. In women they control the output of oestrogen and progesterone and are involved in the ripening each month of a follicle in one of the ovaries, from which an egg is released. We'll not consider male function any further here.

There are two main factors that influence the output of FSH and LH by the pituitary gland, and hence the output of the sex hormones by the ovaries:

1 The release of a hormone from the hypothalamus, called gonadotrophin-releasing hormone (GnRH). This is really the master hormone and it is not important to know much more than this about it in order to understand the menopause, so let's just leave it at that!

2 A feedback effect upon the pituitary gland by the levels of oestrogen and progesterone in the blood. An increase in these hormones dampens down the tendency of the pituitary gland to release FSH and LH, which turns down the output of the hormones by the ovaries. Thus they act as their own controls.

The system is more complicated than this simple description, which is why it is that each month an egg from one of the ovaries is ripened and released under the effect of changing levels of FSH, LH, oestrogen and progesterone. What it is helpful to know is that at the menopause the declining power of the ovaries to produce oestrogen (in particular) means that there is less and less dampening down of the pituitary gland's tendency to release FSH and LH. The typical finding in the blood of a woman who is well into the menopause is therefore that she has high levels of FSH and LH. This is perfectly normal.

Hormone tests

There is much variation in the blood FSH and LH levels prior to the menopause and the large rise is seen only after the menopause is fully established. This means we can't use measurements of LH and FSH to tell us what stage a woman might be along the road to being fully menopausal. That's a pity because, as was mentioned earlier, an easy blood test would be handy from several points of view. So, although high FSH and LH levels confirm the menopause they don't add much to the knowledge you already have if your periods have stopped for

Figure 1: Diagram of feedback control of ovaries by LH and FSH release from the pituitary gland

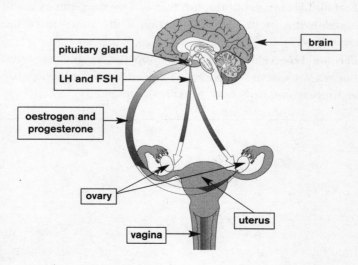

several months or longer. If, however, a woman has had her uterus removed (for example if she's had a lot of trouble from heavy periods) prior to the menopause, then she obviously can't use the absence of periods as a guide to when the menopause has been reached. In her circumstances a blood test showing a rise in the LH and FSH levels is very useful as an indicator that she is menopausal.

LH and FSH levels fall during the use of hormone replacement therapy as these contain oestrogen (and usually progesterone) in sufficient amounts to dampen the release of LH and FSH from the pituitary gland. The system of control and release of the sex hormones is shown in figure 1.

Key Points

- Oestrogen and progesterone are the main sex hormones produced by women, and are manufactured mainly by the ovaries.
- FSH and LH are the hormones released by the pituitary gland beneath the brain and which control the function of the ovaries.
- FSH and LH levels rise after the menopause has fully occurred but we don't have reliable tests that can say if the menopause is approaching or is only partially complete.

Chapter 3

Effects of the Menopause

Knowing a bit about the effects of the sex hormones on the various tissues of the body makes it easier to understand what happens in the menopause when the hormone levels fall. Progesterone generally has a supportive role to oestrogen, which is the main player. Next we'll describe these effects and what they mean in practice when the menopause comes along.

Uterus and vagina

PRE-MENOPAUSE
At puberty the uterus and vagina enlarge under the influence of oestrogen and the lining of the vagina changes to a type that is resistant to trauma. Under the influence of oestrogen the cells of the vaginal lining support the growth of helpful bacteria called lactobacillus, which

produce lactic acid. This has anti-bacterial effects and thus helps reduce the likelihood of vaginal infections. The increased vaginal secretions that occur as a result of sexual arousal and which aid lubrication of the vagina during intercourse are oestrogen-dependent.

Oestrogen has a role in maintaining the strength of the muscles that support the vagina and bladder. The cyclical release of oestrogen and progesterone during the menstrual cycle are the main influences upon the build-up of the uterine lining each month and its shedding at menstruation if pregnancy does not occur.

POST-MENOPAUSE

The vaginal lining becomes thinner and the supporting tissues around it become less elastic. Combined with the fall in vaginal secretions during intercourse, sex can become painful due to vaginal dryness and loss of vaginal relaxation. Bleeding during intercourse may arise, and should be checked to exclude other causes. The lining cells secrete less lactic acid, so the vaginal environment becomes less harsh to bacteria and infection becomes more common. Irritation and itching are common.

Weakness of the muscles that support the bladder and vagina (the pelvic floor muscles) can lead to a dropping down sensation or even a prolapse – in which the internal lining of the vagina and the neck of the womb can appear at the vaginal entrance on standing up or straining. Pelvic floor weakness is worsened in a woman who is overweight and is more likely if she has a history of difficult vaginal delivery.

Bladder

PRE-MENOPAUSE

Oestrogen also helps maintain the strength of the 'valve' muscles that close the bladder when not passing urine (these are called the sphincter muscles). Infections of the urine are common in young women and the symptoms of cystitis will be familiar to many readers. The presence of bacteria in the urine does not always give rise to symptoms though, and 5–10 per cent of pre-menopausal women have 'symptomless bacteriuria' as it's called.

POST-MENOPAUSE
Through the weakening of the pelvic floor and the bladder sphincter a lack of oestrogen increases the likelihood of bacteria entering the bladder. Older women are more likely to have bacteria in the urine and to have symptoms of a urine infection as a result. Weakness of the sphincter or of the pelvic floor increases the chance of being incontinent of urine.

Breasts

Oestrogen stimulates the growth of the breasts, of the milk-producing tissues and ducts and deposits fat in the breast. (It is another hormone, prolactin, which completes the job of making the breasts produce milk. Prolactin is released in increasing amounts by the pituitary gland during the course of pregnancy.) Progesterone stimulates breast tissue growth in the long term but also tends to make the breasts swell on a short-term basis. This is largely due to fluid retention. The naturally high progesterone levels of the second half of a woman's monthly cycle are one of the main reasons why the breasts may feel full and tender before a period.

Oestrogen and progesterone have complex actions on the rates at which new breast cells are normally manufactured. In very general terms oestrogen stimulates the growth of new cells whereas progesterone dampens this process down. This is particularly relevant to the use of HRT in post-menopausal women and is explored in more detail in chapter 6.

Bones

The bones of the skeleton are not just struts that stop us collapsing in a heap. They are very active tissues, continually in a state of repair and remodelling. There are specialised cells throughout bone that are designed to break bone down into its component substances and other cells that take these materials and build new bone again. The balance between the formation of new bone and the absorption of formed bone is a fine one that can change dramatically for many reasons. Following a fracture the manufacturing cells go into overdrive to unite the broken ends with a bridge of new bone. Bone is also capable of adapting over time to increased loads. Thus one sees a thickening of the arm bones in someone used to heavy manual labour. Conversely a prolonged period of inactivity causes a drift downwards in bone strength, especially in the weight-bearing parts of the skeleton.

There are also marked changes in bone activity at puberty. Oestrogen stimulates those cells that manufacture new bone, thus accounting for the growth spurt that often makes adolescent girls taller than their male peers for a few years. However, oestrogen also speeds the closure of the growing part of the long bones such as the femur in the leg. The eventual length of a bone is determined mainly by how long it continues to actively lay down new bone at each end. In girls the growing zone shuts down sooner than in boys, who therefore go on to generally become taller than girls. In the post-menopausal woman the loss of oestrogen stimulation of the bone manufacturing cells means that the bone-absorbing cells win out. This can lead to the weak bone condition called osteoporosis, which is explained in greater detail in chapter 7.

Cardiovascular system

The condition of 'hardening of the arteries' is one of the main problems that commonly affect Western populations. In this condition, properly known as atherosclerosis (or arteriosclerosis), the lining of the arteries becomes thicker, which narrows their internal width and so reduces the flow of blood through them. In addition, the artery lining becomes unstable and prone to causing the clotting of blood over the most unstable parts. If an artery affected by atherosclerosis leading to the heart muscle or to the brain suddenly becomes blocked by a clot then a heart attack or stroke commonly results.

EFFECT OF THE MENOPAUSE ON CARDIOVASCULAR DISEASE

Both men and women develop atherosclerosis and are more likely to do so if they have other 'risk factors' present. These include high blood pressure, smoking, being overweight or diabetic or having a high cholesterol level in the blood. The difference is that men who develop atherosclerosis do so at a younger age than women. This appears to be because of the protective effects of oestrogen in the arteries of pre-menopausal women. Oestrogen acts against the changes that lead to thickening of the artery wall, encourages arteries not to go into spasm and reduces the tendency of blood to clot within arteries. All of these effects reduce the incidence of heart attacks and strokes in pre-menopausal women. Following the menopause women gradually, over a period of several years, begin to show the same rate of cardiovascular disease as men.

Until very recently one of the accepted benefits of using HRT in post-menopausal women was to offer protection against the development of cardiovascular disease. Several recent major studies of HRT have cast doubt on this. In addition, oestrogen treatment is already known to increase the risk of developing clots in the veins (thrombosis). This, and greater detail on the cardiovascular system, are dealt with further in chapter 6, where the pros and cons of HRT are discussed.

Fat, protein and metabolism

Protein is the main constituent of muscle. Oestrogen has a weak positive effect on the growth of protein but is much weaker in this respect than the effect of testosterone in males. Most women will, however, rue the fact that oestrogen is good at promoting the deposition of fat, although it is the oestrogen effect on body fat, especially in the buttocks and thighs, that gives rise to the female shape. There are small and generally unremarkable differences before and after the menopause in the protein and fat make-up of any particular individual that one could put down to the hormone changes on their own. Other factors such as diet, body weight and the level of exercise have a more obvious impact.

'Metabolism' is the general term for all the processes of life put together. In other words this is the energy usage of the body. The higher your metabolism, the greater is the rate at which you consume calories. A high 'metabolic rate' is therefore typical of someone who is engaged in strenuous physical activity. This rate then drops down to a basic level when they rest, although the more muscle someone has the higher is their resting metabolic rate. Someone with a high resting metabolic rate tends to burn off calories more easily than another person with a lower rate. Oestrogen has a positive effect upon metabolism, but only about a third as much as testosterone does. After the menopause there is therefore a drop in metabolism, which can contribute to weight gain. As with fat and protein make-up, however, general lifestyle factors have the most effect on metabolism.

Skin

The effect of oestrogen on skin is to make it soft and smooth. It also increases the blood supply to the skin, making it generally warmer than in men.

TEMPERATURE REGULATION

One of the commonest symptoms of the menopause is 'hot flushes'. Principally these are caused by excessive opening-up of the small blood vessels within the skin, called the capillaries. The commonest place for this to occur is in the upper body, particularly the face and neck region. It's not known exactly why the drop in oestrogen causes hot flushes to occur but it may be due to malfunction of the region within the hypothalamus of the brain that regulates body temperature. Normally the rate of blood flow through the skin is one of the important means we have of maintaining an even body temperature. When we get too hot a rise in blood temperature is detected by the hypothalamus, which sends signals out through the nervous system to the capillaries of the skin, causing them to widen. The increased flow of blood to the skin, along with the sweating process, radiates excess heat away. In cold weather the capillaries are signalled to close, so conserving heat by directing blood away from the skin.

Hot flushes possibly occur because of erroneous signals from the hypothalamus, causing capillary opening when there is no other need for it. Similar wrong signals tell the sweat glands to go into action inappropriately, as flushes and sweats usually go hand in hand. As is described in the paragraph below on the psychological effects of the sex hormones, oestrogen is known to have an influence upon the brain's internal chemistry, and this may be the link that explains why flushes happen.

Sleep

Partly because sweats can be worse at night, but also because of direct effects of oestrogen on brain chemistry, sleep disturbance is a common problem of the menopause. All patterns of abnormal sleep occur: difficulty in getting to sleep, frequent wakening (sometimes drenched in sweat) and early morning wakening with an inability to get back to sleep. All this causes daytime fatigue, lack of concentration and can make you feel down. Early morning wakening is a pattern of sleep disturbance that is also commonly seen in depression, which is another of the links that menopause has with mood.

Psychological effects

Mood is a complex aspect of our behaviour that is not amenable to easy explanations. This is probably one of the main reasons why it is not possible to give a neat summary of the effects that the sex hormones have on any individual's mood. Certainly there is plenty of evidence to show that there is a relationship but it is not a straightforward one.

PRE-MENOPAUSE

Pre-menstrual syndrome, in which mood can fluctuate before a period (and which may be accompanied by other symptoms such as weight gain and bloating) affects between 30 per cent and 80 per cent of women, depending on how it is defined and researched. It has long been the subject of different types of hormonal treatment, but with mostly disappointing results.

It is very likely that sex hormones have a significant effect on mood (both up and down) but we don't have tests that show the link. Measurements of blood levels of the sex hormones do not relate directly to whether a woman will be feeling happy, sad or indifferent at the time, which probably means: a) that the effects of the sex hormones on mood occur over long time scales and are therefore less dependent on the day-to-day changes in blood hormone levels that one can detect; b) it's not the blood level of hormones that's important but the brain levels, which can't be measured.

Perhaps most important is the fact that mood can change in response to such a wide range of influences. Relationships, work and family stresses, general health issues, financial problems and so on all form part of the equation. Each of us has our own set of circumstances to deal with, our own range of emotional reactions and a unique personality. In the face of so many different factors one can only make general observations on the effects on mood of hormone changes.

Given these limitations, however, there is some evidence that shows oestrogen to have mood elevating properties whereas progesterone may lower mood. This may occur through alterations within the brain of the amount of chemical 'messenger' molecules. These are the substances the brain and nervous system uses to relay signals from one cell to the next. Serotonin is one of these, lower amounts of which are found in depression. Oestrogen elevates the brain serotonin level whereas progesterone lowers it, thus possibly explaining one mechanism of how these hormones influence mood.

POST-MENOPAUSE

Given that the sex hormones influence mood it could be expected that at the menopause depression might be more commonly observed. This has been the subject of study and debate for years and experts disagree about whether it is really the case.

Some studies in women who had their ovaries removed surgically and therefore who suffered an abrupt, artificial menopause (often called a 'surgical menopause' in medical circles) showed that they did have a higher risk of developing depression after the operation. Of those women who had a natural menopause those with a long transition time from regular periods to the menopause (i.e. with a long climacteric) were also more likely to become depressed. This may relate to the fact that they had more in the way of fluctuating oestrogen levels for a long time and that this had an adverse effect on mood. Women with a past history of pre-menstrual syndrome or of post-natal depression (depression following giving birth) are also at slightly higher risk of developing menopause-related depression.

Depression is itself a common problem in men and women, although more so in women. Some studies suggest an antidepressant effect for oestrogen replacement therapy but if depression does sometimes arise as a result of the menopause it looks and feels the same as depression from any other cause. One can't therefore say for certain that HRT will help if a woman becomes depressed at this time, but it might and is therefore an option to be borne in mind.

LIFE ADJUSTMENT

The menopause is a time of psychological as well as physical change. Leaving behind the need for contraception may be welcome enough, but loss of the ability to have a child can be harder to take. Our society tends to have a negative view of the menopause – it's often the butt of jokes and being told you're 'menopausal' is not often meant as a compliment. You don't need to look far to find examples of how youthfulness is valued but getting older is treated like the plague. We don't have a culture of respect for older people and if you are thought of as a burden to others you are not going to feel good about yourself.

For a host of reasons, therefore, the menopause can be accompanied by feelings of unworthiness or unattractiveness and a drop in self-esteem. Words alone can't put that right and society's not going to change in a hurry either but we can work on our own attitudes and expectations. Instead of chasing past youth we should instead be looking at what opportunities there are when we're older. The majority of women reaching the menopause nowadays can look forward to as much as 25 to 30 more years of good quality life and some will live way past that. Looked at in that way the menopause is no reason to be hanging up your spurs. Even if we have fewer physical abilities than when young, we've got more time on our hands plus the experience and wisdom to use it better when we get old. Aging comes naturally, but accepting it usually requires a bit of work.

Sexuality

Just as mood is the result of complex interconnected factors, so too is human sexuality and sexual function. The relationship between sexual problems, the menopause, aging and hormone influences has not been particularly well studied. The information we do have shows that for women in the 45–55 age range a decline in sexual interest is significantly associated with the natural menopause, with a decrease in general well-being, with a loss of employment and with the presence of bothersome symptoms such as vaginal dryness or pain during intercourse. This, of course, is very much as you would expect. Sexual interest and function are sensitive to factors that influence a person's general health status and their psychological and social circumstances. A new partner, for example, may be one of the commoner reasons for a mid-life return of sexual interest. A drop in the frequency of sexual intercourse in a loving relationship may simply reflect the fact that partners are happy spending time in each other's company but that their mutual interest in sex is less than it used to be.

Sexual problems tend to feature fairly commonly among those described by women seeking advice and help with the menopause but hormone deficiency rarely covers all the causes. Certainly if physical problems such as vaginal dryness are prominent then relief of those with treatment can go a long way to restoring a woman's ability to enjoy sex. But there is much more to sexual enjoyment than the act itself and hormones are no substitute for care and intimacy in a person's life. The male partners of women in this age group perhaps need to remember this!

Not a disease

The aim of this chapter has been to cover the main aspects of the biology of the menopause: how it affects the body, the mind and our behaviour. The purpose of this nuts and bolts approach has been to aid understanding, and not to make the process look like an obstacle course fraught with problems! Most women do not experience all of these symptoms to a major degree and many have little trouble with the menopause. The majority recognise that quite a few symptoms strike a chord with them, but don't necessarily see them as hard to live with, nor do they necessarily want treatment for them. Often a bit of understanding from those around them, accompanied by some give and take, is all they are asking for. We said at the beginning that the menopause is a natural part of life, and is not a disease. Living with it isn't an option – it has to be done – so the next chapter looks at the general things you can do to cope with it better.

Key Points

- Oestrogen deficiency is the main cause of the hormone-related effects of the menopause, with progesterone deficiency of secondary importance.
- Recognised changes occur in virtually every body system as a result of the menopause.
- Of most importance are the effects on the uterus and vagina, breasts, bones and cardiovascular system.
- The menopause can cause significant mood changes but on its own probably does not cause serious mental ill health.

Chapter 4

Coping with the Menopause

A healthy lifestyle

A lot of the time we spend as adults is not focussed on keeping healthy. The statistics for the increasing numbers of people developing obesity, high blood pressure, heart disease, diabetes and many types of cancer speak volumes about our present trend towards becoming a nation populated mostly by unfit and overweight people. The only way we can avoid becoming part of this stereotype is to get a grip on our own lives and do something about it. Most of the things you can do about the menopause are the same things that will improve your general health. As we said earlier, the menopause is a good time to take stock of our lifestyle and to make improvements.

The concept of a 'one size fits all' approach to keeping healthy is an important one. There has been too much tendency over the years to put health issues into boxes and for advice to be fragmented into separate categories. Thus people with high blood pressure have been told to keep to a low salt diet, those with high cholesterol levels to cut down on their fat intake, people with diabetes to watch the calories and the sugar intake. The list goes on and on.

Although there can be a need for individual tailoring of lifestyle changes, most of what is good for us in terms of improving blood pressure control, cholesterol levels or whatever else is the same advice as we all ought to follow anyway. A healthy balanced diet, avoidance of smoking and excess alcohol intake, regular exercise, decent sleep and some leisure time are effective remedies for many of life's ills, and reduce the chances of developing many of the medical problems attached to the Western way of life. The menopause can be tackled in the same way.

There is something of an explosion going on in non drug-related ways to treat the menopause, for good reasons. There have always been people, including some medical authorities, who doubted the benefits of HRT and these misgivings have been brought to the fore by the results of some recent medical trials. The move away from drug treatments has, however, been going on for a long time and mirrors the huge expansion in interest in complementary medical treatments over the past ten to 20 years. People are no longer happy to blandly accept the medicines their doctor prescribes without knowing more about the side effects of those treatments. They also want to know more about how they can help themselves. That's a good thing, although we've a long way to go before we see people from all sections of society able and willing to look after themselves better. As you are interested enough to read this book it's very likely that you are in the group that wishes to make the right moves.

HELPING YOURSELF

There are four broad areas where you can take action on your own behalf to cope with the menopause:

1 information and understanding;
2 diet and nutrition, including vitamin and mineral supplements;
3 exercise and other lifestyle modifications;
4 herbal remedies and complementary medicine.

Information gathering and understanding

That's what you're doing right now, and hopefully this book will be helpful in giving you the necessary facts about the menopause. There are other sources of information and help listed in appendix C. This is a time of uncertainty in medical as well as public circles about the rights and the wrongs of menopause and the conventional treatments for it. A lot of doctors are just as confused as their patients at the moment and it will probably be several years before some of these presently controversial areas are cleared up. In the meantime we can still act on the basis of the best available information along with some common sense. Most of us appreciate that life isn't perfect anyway and that many decisions need to be made on the basis of imperfect knowledge.

Understanding the menopause also helps others around you (who may not be female or if so are not yet at that stage of life!) to appreciate what you are going through. If this book ends up being dog-eared because everyone in your family has read it then well and good.

Knowing what the uses and limitations are of conventional HRT means you will be in a better position than many women currently using it to decide whether to take it or leave it. In the next chapter we also cover the conventional medications that are *not* HRT but which also have potential benefits in the menopause.

Diet and nutrition

Nutrition affects the menopause in three ways:

1 By providing direct symptom relief. The main candidates in this category are natural oestrogens from plant sources, called 'phyto-estrogens'.
2 By reducing the risk of cardiovascular disease and cancer. These are recognised benefits that accompany healthy eating behaviour in all people. In women post-menopause they are particularly important in offsetting the rise in cardiovascular disease that goes with the natural fall in oestrogen.
3 By maintaining or improving bone strength.

1. PHYTOESTROGENS

There is disagreement about whether plant oestrogens have anything more than a 'placebo' effect in the menopause. The placebo effect is the observation that even inert or dummy treatment can seem helpful if the person taking it believes strongly enough that it works.

One of the pointers towards a positive effect from phytoestrogens is that Japanese women are reported to have a low chance of getting hot flushes from the menopause. Their diet is high in phytoestrogens (which are present in high concentration in soy), hence the possible link. Those experts who are not so sure of this point to the possibility that Japanese women perhaps don't complain so much of flushes in surveys.

Part of the difficulty is that phytoestrogens are a diverse and complex family of substances, which have been isolated in over 300 types of plant. The two main subdivisions are known as lignans (present in flaxseed, linseed and whole grain cereals) and isoflavones (present in pulses like soy beans and chick peas and in clovers). Other foodstuffs in which they are found include apples, carrots, coffee, potatoes, yams, bean sprouts, sunflower and sesame seeds, rye and wheat.

It is also difficult to do long-term studies of differences in diet between large numbers of people over several years, as is necessary with a situation such as the menopause, and to be sure that observed differences in the groups of people being studied are all due to what they were eating and not a host of other factors to do with their lifestyle. So although there is some official scepticism over the effectiveness of phytoestrogens it may be impossible to be any more precise. If you are bothered by flushes it is a safe option to increase the amount of phytoestrogens you eat and see if it helps. Although there is some evidence that phytoestrogens have a favourable effect on the levels of fat in the blood and on bone strength this is not certain enough on its own to recommend them. It is possible to buy phyto-estrogens in concentrated capsule form, which may be a convenient way of ensuring an adequate enough intake to convince yourself one way or the other if they help you. The best way though is to increase your dietary intake by choosing foods rich in phytoestrogens, incorporating them more in what you eat. As a bonus you'll benefit from the extra vitamins and other nutrients that real food has and packaged supplements can only vaguely mimic.

2. REDUCING THE RISK OF CARDIOVASCULAR DISEASE AND CANCER

These two areas are now well accepted as places where achievable dietary changes can make an impact on how well and how long all of us live. For the post-menopausal woman, increasingly exposed to developing hardening of the arteries the longer she is past the oestrogen-producing years, this is particularly important. You'll see from what follows that several aspects of generally healthy diets coincide exactly with good advice points we've already mentioned about the menopause.

The main dietary features that raise cardiovascular risk are:

- high intake of saturated (hard) fats, fatty acids, cholesterol and calories;
- low intake of fruit and vegetables (fewer than five portions of fruit and vegetables per day);
- high intake of salt.

A healthy diet is therefore one that:

- is low in fat,
- is low in sugar,
- includes at least five portions of fruit and vegetables every day,
- is high in fibre,
- contains pulses, e.g. beans and lentils,
- is moderate in cereals, bread and potatoes,
- is low in salt.

Fats and fatty acids

Fat is particularly high in calories, so reducing fat intake is a central part of weight-reducing diets. Some fat is, however, essential in our diet. In addition to providing a source of concentrated energy, fats contain the essential fat-soluble vitamins A, D, E and K.

The two main types of fat are 'saturated' and 'unsaturated'. Saturated fats are solid at room temperature and are the more undesirable from the health point of view. They are found mainly in lard, red meat, suet, dripping, eggs and full-fat dairy products. They are also found in hard margarines – which are often used for making cakes, biscuits and pastry. Avoiding these items will reduce your saturated fat intake considerably.

Unsaturated or 'good' fats are generally liquid at room temperature and come from vegetable sources but are also found in oily fish and in soft margarines labelled 'high in polyunsaturates'. These unsaturated fats also contain essential fatty acids that cannot be manufactured by the body and need to be obtained from food. 'Omega-3' and 'omega-6' fatty acids are types found in oily fish and which appear to give additional protection against cardiovascular disease.

Some practical tips regarding dietary fat are:

- Choose lean meat or poultry, removing the excess fat before cooking.
- Try to reduce your intake of dairy products and eat more fat-free or soya-based dairy products.
- Use semi-skimmed or soya milk in your tea and coffee and on your cereal.
- Avoid hard margarines, biscuits and pastries.
- Avoid frying and roasting foods – steam, grill, stir-fry and bake instead.
- Try to eat oily fish 2–3 times a week (herring, mackerel, mullet, salmon, trout, tuna, sardines, anchovies).

Diet and cancer

The body constantly reacts with oxygen as part of the energy-producing processes of cells. As a consequence of this activity, highly reactive molecules are produced, known as free radicals. These interact with other molecules within the cell, which can cause oxidative damage to proteins, cell membranes and genes. This damage has been implicated in the cause of many diseases including cancers and has an impact on the body's aging process.

Antioxidants are substances that neutralise free radicals and the body produces an armoury of them to defend itself. The metabolic processes that produce antioxidants are controlled and influenced by an individual's genetic make-up and the extra environmental factors (such as diet, smoking and pollution) to which your body is exposed. Unfortunately, changes in our lifestyles, which include more environmental pollution and less quality in our diets, mean that we are exposed to more free radicals than ever before. Our internal production of antioxidants is insufficient to neutralise and scavenge all the free radicals but there is an abundant supply of antioxidants in a wide variety of foods. By increasing our dietary intake of antioxidants, we can help our body to defend itself.

Examples of food-based antioxidants include:

- The vitamins (vitamin E, vitamin C, and beta-carotene).
- The trace elements that are components of antioxidant enzymes (including selenium, copper, zinc and manganese).
- Some non-nutrients such as ubiquinone (coenzyme Q), which is sometimes used as an 'energy booster'. Phytoestrogens are themselves antioxidants.
- Tomatoes contain a pigment, lycopene, which is responsible for the red colour but is also a powerful antioxidant. Tomatoes in all their forms are the major source of lycopene and include tomato products like canned tomatoes, tomato soup, tomato juice and even ketchup. Lycopene is also highly concentrated in watermelon.
- Oranges, grapefruit, lemons and limes possess many natural substances that appear to be important in disease protection. Together these 'phytochemicals' act more powerfully than if they were given separately. It's always better to eat the fruit whole in its natural form, as some of the potency is lost when the juice is extracted.
- Black tea, green tea and oolong teas have antioxidant properties. All three varieties come from the plant called *Camellia sinensis*. Common brands of black tea do contain antioxidants, but the most potent is green tea (jasmine tea), which contains the antioxidant catechin. Oolong tea has only 40 per cent as much of the antioxidants found in green tea and black tea has only 10 per cent as much. When green tea is processed (baked and fermented) to make black tea, some of the catechins are destroyed.
- Beta-carotene is an orange pigment isolated from carrots 150 years ago. It is found concentrated in deep orange and green vegetables

(the green chlorophyll covers up the orange pigment). Carrots also contain phytoestrogens.

3. DIET AND BONE HEALTH

A good calcium intake is essential throughout life for healthy bones and there is good evidence that the adequacy of a child's diet at least partially determines their osteoporosis risk in adulthood. Although dairy products are high in calcium they are not the only source. Non-dairy food sources include: nuts and pulses (almonds, Brazil nuts, hazelnuts, sesame seeds), green leafy vegetables (broccoli, spinach, watercress, curly kale), dried fruits (apricots, dates, figs, prunes), fish (mackerel, pilchards, salmon, sardines), tofu and various calcium-fortified foods.

The daily intake of calcium required by an adult is around 800 milligrams. On average 250ml or half a pint of cow's milk or 150g/5oz of yoghurt contains 300 milligrams of calcium and low-fat dairy products contain the same amount of calcium as higher fat varieties. Calcium supplements can be bought and there are several types available on prescription if someone's dietary intake is low or marginal.

Vitamin D has a potent effect on increasing the absorption of calcium from the diet and is directly involved in controlling bone growth and repair. Actually vitamin D is not the active form of the substance, which is manufactured within the body by a series of steps, one of which requires ultra-violet light on the skin. Adequate exposure to sunlight is therefore another essential requirement for healthy bones. Good sources of vitamin D include: butter, cheese, cod liver oil, eggs, liver, margarine, mackerel and other oily fish, yoghurt.

Magnesium is important in a range of metabolic processes and adequate amounts are necessary for calcium to be properly utilised. Good food sources are similar to those for calcium, as well as bananas, brown rice, courgettes, lean meat, parsnips, sweetcorn, wholemeal bread and pasta.

Several other vitamins and trace elements are important for bone health and although calcium and vitamin D supplements are quite often used to protect against developing osteoporosis, especially in the elderly, it may also be helpful to take a general multivitamin preparation too. More information on osteoporosis is in chapter 7.

Nutritional supplements

Some of these have already been mentioned and many are antioxidants. With the exception of phytoestrogen supplements, most are not specifically effective for the menopause but instead are beneficial to health in general.

Strictly speaking it should not be necessary for someone taking a good balanced diet to need vitamin and mineral supplements – after all human beings have managed to survive for millions of years without them. Many surveys, however, point to the inadequacy of the diet that many Britons eat. Whether those people with deficient diets are the same as those who buy vitamin supplements is a moot point, but the fact remains that these additives are part of a multi-million pound industry that is increasingly popular. There are lots of uncertainties surrounding nutritional supplements, including how one decides on which ones to use, who will benefit most, what the correct doses are and, increasingly, what they all do together when taken in amounts that are greater than normally found in the human diet. It won't be possible to answer these questions here either. Natural sources are almost always better than artificial ones, so where possible we mention those foods that are particularly rich in the most beneficial vitamins and minerals.

B VITAMINS AND FOLIC ACID

The many different vitamins classified under this group are essential for the biochemical functioning of cells and the production of blood by the bone marrow. In the context of cardiovascular disease, inadequate dietary amounts of these items leads to a build-up in the blood of a substance called homocysteine, which is capable of damaging the lining of arteries. It's thought that oestrogen plays a role in keeping homocysteine low in pre-menopausal women, partly explaining why they are less likely to have cardiovascular disease.

Vitamin B6 has been used over the years as a treatment for pre-menstrual syndrome, but not with great results. It's sometimes recommended for low mood around the time of the menopause but does not have any definite evidence supporting this use.

Sources of B vitamins include: asparagus, bananas, broccoli, brown rice, cheese, dried apricots and figs, eggs, fish, nuts, poultry, pulses, red meat, spinach, wheat germ, wholegrain cereals, yeast extract (e.g. Marmite), yoghurt. Vegetarians who eat eggs and dairy produce will obtain sufficient amounts of vitamin B12 from their diet but vegans may need to take a supplement.

Folic acid occurs naturally in most foods although often in small amounts. Many foods are now fortified with folic acid and supplements are given to mothers in early pregnancy (or before they conceive), as folic acid reduces the chance of spina bifida occurring in the baby.

The greatest concentration of folic acid is found in liver. Other good sources are: asparagus, avocados, beef, broccoli, citrus fruits, curly kale, dried beans and peas, lamb, pork, Savoy cabbage, spinach, tomatoes, turnip, wheat germ (wholemeal bread and cereals), other wholegrain products such as pasta and brown rice.

VITAMIN E

This is a powerful antioxidant and is thought to play an important part in reducing cardiovascular disease and fighting cancer. It also lowers blood fat levels. Some European studies have suggested that a low level of vitamin E is actually a better predictor of heart disease than raised cholesterol or blood pressure. It's also said to have some ability to reduce hot flushes.

Good sources are: avocados, blackberries, Brussels sprouts, corn oil, mackerel, mangoes, nuts, olive oil, tomatoes, salmon, soft margarine, spinach, sunflower oil, sweet potatoes, watercress, wheat germ and wholegrain cereal.

IPRIFLAVONE

This is a synthetically produced phytoestrogen increasingly popular as a supplement to prevent osteoporosis. There is some research work, mostly from Japan, suggesting it is effective for this.

Exercise and other lifestyle modifications

EXERCISE

Technology, in the form of motorised transport, has removed the need for us to expend energy getting from A to B. We no longer have to forage for food – a glide along the aisles of the local supermarket is the closest we come to that activity now. Television and computer games allow us to occupy our minds without engaging our bodies. All of these activities run counter to the way we are designed to work in a biological sense and have been in the habit of living for thousands of years. The relationship between inactivity and cardiovascular risk was observed over 50 years ago, in the observational studies comparing the rate of heart disease between London bus drivers and their conductor colleagues. The epidemics of diabetes and obesity have occurred in only the past 25 years, coincident with the rise of the leisure age. The linkage is clear.

The evidence supporting the health benefits of exercise is now overwhelming. In addition to major reductions in coronary heart disease regular moderately intense physical activity reduces blood pressure and cholesterol levels, lowers the occurrence of obesity, diabetes, cancer of the colon and the breast and increases psychological well-being. Particularly relevant to the menopause is that regular exercise protects against osteoporosis (it does so for men too, and we've given some space to the 'male menopause' in chapter 9). Of all the stress-busting treatments that we undoubtedly need in this day and age, nothing is as effective or as good for you as a long walk. Particularly good news for those people already suffering from signs of cardio-vascular disease is that they benefit proportionately more from physical activity compared to others at lower risk.

For those who've been in the habit of taking regular exercise, whether running or anything else, it will be natural to keep on going into a ripe old age. However, a very large proportion of the population of all ages presently takes little or no significant regular exercise. If you are one of them then the good news is that you can get back into exercise mode quite rapidly by applying a bit of common sense. Once you do you'll be improving your health in just about every possible way.

Physical activity needs to be maintained in order to be of most benefit. Several studies have confirmed that individuals have a reduced coronary heart disease risk during the periods of life when they are active, but if they then adopt a sedentary lifestyle their risk goes up. The reverse is also true.

Walking is in many ways the ideal form of exercise. It can be undertaken by most people and started at a modest level appropriate for someone who's been out of the exercise habit for a long time. It doesn't need expensive equipment and can be as social or as private as you want it to be. Brisk walking is good aerobic exercise that doesn't jar the joints too much and injuries when walking are rare. Cycling is also suitable for a wide range of people and can often be incorporated easily into daily living. Its benefits are staggering. Cycling for one hour or for 25 miles per week was associated with a 50 per cent reduction in risk of dying *from all causes* over a 10-year follow-up period in one study.

The recommended amount of exercise that achieves health improvement is 30 minutes of brisk walking (or similar exercise) on five or six days a week. This is a slight shift away from earlier advice that promoted more vigorous, sustained activity designed to improve heart and lung function and fitness. Moderate activity, as currently recommended, also improves fitness but at a slower rate and to a lower level. From a public health perspective this is important as it makes clear that worthwhile exercise is feasible and sustainable for the vast majority of people.

Electronic gadgets to count the number of steps you take are cheap and can be quite revealing, as well as motivating. A target of 10,000 steps daily should be your eventual aim – the average office day produces 3,000 steps. The most important factor is to repeat the exercise frequently and build up gradually to a long-term change in your routine.

Modifying your routine can help work some more exercise in without much effort. Leaving the car at home for short journeys or using a bicycle instead are obvious enough. Getting off the bus or tube a stop before your destination is easy. Shunning the lift and using the stairs should be your habit. Swimming is an excellent all-round form of exercise that is suitable for almost everyone to undertake. Like walking, you can pace it to suit yourself. If you can't swim, then now is an excellent time to think about getting some lessons!

All of these actions and more are possible. The real block to getting exercise is not generally a physical one or even because of a lack of somewhere nice to walk – although it certainly helps. Most of the block is psychological. Coming home from a busy day you'll perhaps be in the habit of flopping into a chair, and once you're there you'll probably not be keen to get up again. However this is a good time to have a walk instead. You'll clear your mind as well as your arteries, be less likely to reach for a drink and will probably eat less when you sit down to your evening meal.

Like a rusty flywheel, it might be hard to get started but once you are in exercise mode you'll tend to keep it going. You'll find that your mood and energy levels improve, that you can think more clearly and that you feel less strung out. Both in the short and the long term exercise will reduce the impact of the menopause on your mind and your body.

ALCOHOL

Consuming a small amount of alcohol daily (up to two standard units) appears to have a beneficial effect upon our arteries and helps stop them clogging up. There are many possible explanations for this, but among the most likely are that compounds within some alcoholic drinks, particularly red wine, are also effective antioxidants that can neutralise free radical molecules. However, the effects rapidly turn from beneficial to harmful when higher levels of alcohol are consumed. Men and women who have a high alcohol intake have a higher risk of developing osteoporosis.

The usual recommended maximum consumption of alcohol per week is:

- 21 units for women,
- 28 units of alcohol for men

but many experts believe that more modest levels are safer:

- 14 units per week for women,
- 21 units per week for men.

A unit of alcohol is:

- 250ml (½ pint) of ordinary strength beer/lager,
- 1 glass (125ml/4 fl oz) of wine,
- 1 pub measure of sherry/vermouth (1.5oz),
- 1 pub measure of spirits (1.5oz).

Bear in mind that unmeasured home-poured spirit drinks will usually be generous, so get into the habit of using a spirit measure and sticking to it!

RELAXATION TIME

One of the reasons why getting out for a walk helps you feel better is that it usually means taking some time out to do it. Most of us slide into the situation where we never seem to have any time for ourselves. 'Stress' is hard to define but we all know what it means and nobody denies that modern day living is stressful. We all need some time off now and again but unless you are very lucky, other people won't make your breaks for you! Taking a break to watch TV, read the paper, do some gardening or just stare at the ceiling won't make any difference to the number of jobs on your list. Admittedly this is a general lifestyle issue and not one limited to the menopause. But as we're looking at the menopause in its proper position as part of your life and not as a bolt-on attachment then if you've spent the first four or five decades of your life chasing other people's deadlines, make a resolution now to start looking after number one a bit more.

Simple relaxation techniques are easy to learn and can be remarkably effective at defusing stress. For example, just sit down in a quiet room (if available!) and deliberately relax every muscle in your body, consciously going through every region from the top of your head to the tips of your toes. Control your breathing as you do so and try to clear your mind of thoughts. Maintain the relaxed state for a few minutes at least before going about your business again and you'll find that you can tackle the next problem more easily. If you don't think it will help, try it and see but remember not to rush it.

Use of herbal medicines and complementary treatments

The increase in interest in these forms of therapy shows no sign of slowing down. The menopause is a major reason for women to try them out, even if they've never done so for any other reason before. Herbal medicines are generally seen as natural, safe, mild and more acceptable than 'drugs'. Without wishing to deny that view, it's prudent to remember that this is not always so. Many herbal remedies are relatively untested for effect and the purity, strength and safety of some is very difficult to be sure of. The testing process for herbal medicines is much less stringent than that for prescription medicines. The message here, therefore, is that if you wish to use herbal preparations (and there's plenty of cause to think that they can be helpful in the menopause) then make sure you get them from a reliable source.

Similarly there are all sorts of alternative medical practitioners around and the level of training and fitness to practise of many of them can be open to question. There are, however, ways of checking that a therapist is trained or qualified in many of the popular alternative medical therapies and some relevant contact numbers for the professional or governing bodies of these are listed in appendix C.

Conventional medical attitudes to herbal medicines and complementary treatments are changing for the better but there are still plenty of people around with entrenched views. There are the devotees of 'evidence-based medicine' who can't find the academic studies that show these therapies work better than placebo. There are also the many millions of satisfied users of such treatments who rightly have a better opinion of themselves than as simply gullible consumers or the victims of faddism.

In contrast to the vast resources of the conventional pharmaceutical industry, which spends billions of pounds annually on drug research, the amount of funding that goes into complementary research is tiny. There is little or no money to be made, in drug industry terms, in finding out if a particular type of herb is useful in treating a condition because the treatment could not be patented or commercialised.

There is a large body of medical literature on complementary treatments but it will never be comparable, either in quality or quantity, to 'conventional' treatments. For some doctors, and patients, that means that complementary medicine is a no-go area. For others willing to live with the fact that life isn't perfect then there is much to be gained from them.

Herbal treatments

Herbs generally contain more than one active constituent, which can vary considerably in its concentration depending on the part of the plant used, the season of the year when it is harvested and the growing conditions of the soil, etc. For this reason, the same plant can often have more than one use. Thousands of such compounds have been catalogued and many have been studied in detail.

Many of the ways in which herbal treatments are used are dictated by culture or by systems of practice that go back hundreds if not thousands of years. Thus one sees different treatments and methods used in India compared to China or Europe. Although some women can afford the cost of consulting a trained herbalist privately in the UK, most have to rely upon what they can get in the pharmacy or health shop. The purists may say that this is a poor second best because such treatments need to be tailored to the individual, but that's a restriction that most of us just have to live with. Bearing in mind, therefore, that the amount of evidence supporting their effectiveness is usually lightweight or absent, and that choosing remedies isn't the same as choosing the ingredients for a recipe, then there is little to be lost by trying them out on yourself. At the risk of stating the obvious, if you are tempted to dig over a corner of your garden and plant a few for your own use – don't! Many herbal plants are potentially poisonous unless they are prepared in the correct way.

BLACK COHOSH (*CIMICIFUGA RACEMOSA*)

This is probably the most popular single herbal remedy for the menopause. Its alternative names such as black snakeroot, rattlehead and squaw root derive from its North American origins and it has been in use for hundreds of years as a treatment for painful periods, irregular menstruation or other problems such as headaches, rheumatism and colds. There are many active compounds present in the herb, including phytoestrogens, vitamin C, beta-carotene and trace metals. It's generally thought that it works through a mild oestrogen-like activity. Its usefulness is for hot flushes and headaches, irritability, palpitations and vaginal dryness. It appears to be safe in long-term use.

CHASTE TREE (*VITEX AGNUS CASTUS*)

The common name of this Mediterranean shrub derives from its traditional use as a dampener of the libido. It has been used for the relief of pre-menstrual symptoms such as breast pain and is also said to relieve menopausal symptoms, although the evidence in this respect is scant.

WILD YAM (SWEET POTATO) AND LIQUORICE

Yams are root vegetables now commonly available in the supermarkets. Liquorice is made from the long snake-like root of *Glycyrrhiza glabra*. Both have mild oestrogen- and progesterone-like qualities. Liquorice also contains a substance that can raise the blood pressure, although you need to take a lot of it for that to happen. Some studies using combinations of black cohosh, liquorice, chaste tree and wild yam produced good results for menopausal symptom relief.

ST JOHN'S WORT (*HYPERICUM PERFORATUM*)

This is a perennial plant about 45cm high with a bare trunk and yellow flowers, which grows mainly in Europe, Asia and North America. The deep green leaves contain oil glands, which let through light and give the appearance of perforations – hence its name. Its use in herb lore goes back hundreds of years, as a treatment for wounds and for warding off witches! All growing parts of the plant above the soil are used to manufacture a crude form of the herb called hypericum extract, which is known to contain a range of active ingredients. The precise amounts of these compounds vary between species and are dependent also upon growing conditions and the time when the plant is harvested.

A study reported in the British Medical Journal in 1999 compared hypericum extract with imipramine (an older type of antidepressant) over a period of eight weeks in people with moderate depression. Hypericum was at least as good as imipramine, and was better tolerated. Hypericum has been used as a herbal treatment for depression, anxiety and sleep disorders for some time in Germany where herbal medicine is more popular than in the UK, but many of the previous research studies investigating its effectiveness have not been of a high scientific standard.

The dose of extract used in this study was 350mg three times daily. Hypericum tablets in the UK contain about 300mg per tablet. Hypericum can clash with other medications including the contraceptive pill and can cause a light-sensitive rash in some people. As with all such remedies it is best to check with the pharmacist if you are going to take it, but on the basis of the available evidence it appears to be a reasonable treatment to try for mild depression, whether or not this is associated with the menopause.

OTHER HERBAL REMEDIES

The list of herbal remedies that have been used for the relief of various menopausal symptoms is a long one and beyond the scope of this book to cover. Brief details of some, including the effects ascribed to them in the herbal literature are:

- *Valerian*: a sedative useful to promote sleep or relieve anxiety and migraine.
- *Ginkgo biloba*: relieves anxiety and depression and improves memory.
- *Motherwort*: a sedative and anxiety reliever.

Complementary treatments

'Complementary' is a better term than 'alternative' for the many forms of therapy, including herbal medicine, that are now so popular as it implies that conventional Western medicine can and should co-exist alongside them. An increasingly high proportion of doctors realise that the medicines and methods they were trained to use are often of little use against the range of problems that human beings can have. Patients are also voting with their feet in large numbers and seeking out complementary practitioners for a variety of reasons. The reticence that some doctors have about such treatments is not all because of closed-mindedness (although that accounts for a fair bit) but is also because of genuine concern that their patients will eschew treatments that they know will work, or will delay seeing them for an accurate diagnosis of something serious, or that they don't like seeing their patients being ripped off. Only rarely are such worries well founded but they shouldn't be ignored.

Even if the problem seems easily to fit with an obvious cause such as the menopause, it is always a good idea to consult your GP first and obtain a good diagnosis of whatever it is that ails you. After that you can have a dialogue about what you will do about it, and if that choice is towards complementary treatments it's to be hoped that your doctor will support that decision. He or she may not have much experience of the other treatments so you may find that you are back on your own resources when it comes to finding a good therapist. Check when possible with the controlling or registering bodies that you are seeing someone who is up to scratch.

The advantages of treatments such as acupuncture, aromatherapy, massage, yoga and so on in terms of the menopause are not well established. Most of these are good at promoting relaxation and general fitness, which is good enough reason to partake as we've already said. Of the complementary treatments we've not yet mentioned, homoeopathy is the main one that deserves a bit more coverage.

Homoeopathy

Homoeopathy has been around for over 200 years and is an 'official' part of NHS treatment. Although there are only a handful of homoeopathic hospitals in the UK (see appendix C) many doctors, particularly GPs, have undertaken some training in it and can offer homoeopathic treatment to their patients. Many homoeopaths work privately, and not all have medical qualifications.

Homoeopathic remedies are made from many materials, but are usually plant-based. Unlike herbal remedies, though, they are extremely dilute. Many conventional doctors remain sceptical of homoeopathy, particularly in view of the very low concentration of 'active ingredient' within the remedies, but many studies do show that it is better than placebo for many conditions, and there is no doubt that it remains very popular. One of the good things about homoeopathic remedies is that they are completely safe, and do not clash with conventional medications.

Homoeopathic remedies need to be tailored to the individual so an off-the-shelf approach may not work. Usually a homeopath will select a small range of particularly chosen preparations that match as many as possible of the symptoms as well as the personality traits of the patient. As with herbal treatments, though, many people will simply wish to try what they can easily buy from the pharmacy or health store. Some preparations contain a mixture of many homoeopathic remedies, which might be a reasonable way of covering lots of options. The following individual remedies may be of most use for menopausal symptoms:

- *Sepia*: hot flushes, fatigue, night sweats, poor sleep.
- *Calcarea carbonica*: daytime flushes, sweats.
- *Lachesis*: flushes, especially about the neck, temperature fluctuations.
- *Phosphorus*: flushes, palpitations, anxiety, dizziness.
- *Sanguinaria*: intense heat, flushes – especially with headaches, pulsating sensations throughout the body.
- *Sulphur*: feeling warm all the time, always sweating.

Complementary versus conventional

Nothing is lost by trying safe complementary treatments for the acute symptoms of the menopause. Whatever the scientific basis may be for or against them, you can make up your own mind if they are doing you any obvious good. However, we also need to consider the longer-term aspects of the menopause and the effects we know it has on the heart and blood vessels and the bones for example. These are hidden effects that don't have any obvious symptoms, or at least not in the early stages. The evidence in favour of using complementary treatments to ward off osteoporosis is not good enough to make recommendations one way or the other for the long term. In the next sections of the book we therefore concentrate on the conventional treatments available and the pros and cons of using them.

Key Points

- Coping with the menopause has a lot in common with coping with life in general.
- Self-help is a very important aspect of menopause treatment, and becoming well informed is the first and most important step in that process.
- Diet and nutrition, exercise and lifestyle modifications can all make a substantial difference to how the menopause affects an individual woman.
- Although the scientific basis for many complementary treatments is weak compared to prescription medicines, they are popular and have an important part to play.

Chapter 5

Medicines for the Menopause

In terms of the number of preparations available most of the conventional treatments in use for the menopause are hormone replacement therapy in one form or another. HRT is, however, not the only important form of treatment to consider. In this chapter we'll deal first with HRT and then move on to the others.

Hormone replacement therapy

There is an obvious logic to the use of hormones to boost the fall in output of the menopausal ovaries. Premarin® was the first available such pharmaceutical and was released in 1942. A mixture of oestrogens (called conjugated oestrogens), it is still in wide use today.

One point to mention in case of confusion is that **progesterone** is the name of the particular hormone produced naturally by the ovary but there are several progesterone-like compounds in use in HRT. The general name for these is **progestogens**. Oestrogen is a bit different as three types are manufactured normally by human beings! We don't need to know more than that, and that the collective name **oestrogens** is used for all of them, including those used in HRT.

EARLY HRT EXPERIENCE

Oestrogen replacement had the desired effect of relieving menopausal symptoms but it was discovered in the 1970s that women using it who still had their womb (i.e. they had not had it removed for some reason like heavy bleeding, for example) had an increased risk of developing cancer of the lining of the womb after some years of oestrogen use. The medical name for the lining of the womb is the endometrium, hence this type of cancer is called endometrial cancer. The reason was traced to the continuous stimulating effect of oestrogen upon the cells of the endometrium.

During the normal menstrual cycle oestrogen waxes and wanes and so too does progesterone. Oestrogen predominates in the first half of the cycle and progesterone in the second. In general terms cancer occurs when a cell runs out of control, duplicating repeatedly without obeying the normal rules that govern cell behaviour. Progesterone appears to have a natural regulating influence on the womb lining cells – it's the brake whereas oestrogen is the accelerator. In the presence of oestrogen but absence of progesterone some womb lining cells are overproduced and over time some eventually lose control and can become cancerous. It was then discovered that by adding progestogen as well as oestrogen to the treatment the problem of endometrial cancer was largely reversed, although not eliminated. (We'll deal in more detail with the risks associated with HRT in the next chapter.)

The use of oestrogen on its own ('unopposed oestrogen') is therefore not safe in women who still have their uterus, no matter when in relation to their menopause they start taking HRT. The usual name for HRT that uses both oestrogen and progestogen is 'combined HRT'.

Conversely, women who have had their uterus removed and who are otherwise suitable to take HRT need only take oestrogen and can dispense with the progestogen.

TYPES OF HORMONES IN USE

The various hormones available today are made using combinations of natural and synthetic chemical processes. Some use soy or yams as source material, others use entirely artificial means to produce them. The oestrogen in Premarin® (and its 'combined' partners Prempak-C® and Premique®) was and still is made by extracting the oestrogens present in the urine of pregnant mares, hence its name.

Drug company chemists have produced a range of oestrogens and progestogens not so much because they think they can do better than nature but more to overcome practical problems associated with getting the hormones into the body where they can do their work. All medicines taken by mouth have to run the gauntlet of being digested by stomach acid and the enzymes of the intestines and they then face being turned into some other chemical by the body's own processing plant; the liver. To get hormones inside tablets to survive these hurdles intact, changes to their chemical nature are made while still preserving the original hormone activity.

The differences in the precise chemical nature of the oestrogens and progestogens used in the various types of HRT does not appear to be important as far as their ability to relieve the symptoms of the menopause is concerned. They all do that very well. Where there may be differences is in their long-term safety. This is another topic that will be covered in the next chapter.

The types of oestrogen and progestogen used in HRT are very similar to those used in the oral contraceptive pill. However, the strength of the oestrogen used in HRT is several times less than that used in the pill. HRT tablets do not give any protection against pregnancy. The issue of what to do about contraception when you are around and about the menopause but not fully past it is dealt with in chapter 10.

Forms of HRT available

Although there are dozens of individual brands of HRT available for a doctor to prescribe they break down into a smaller number of categories:

1 **Local treatments**: oestrogen creams, tablets ('pessaries') or rings inserted high in the vagina which are impregnated with oestrogen that slowly leaks out, for the relief of vaginal symptoms such as dryness, irritation and pain on intercourse.
2 **Oral treatments**: tablets of oestrogen alone or along with pro-gesterone in combined HRT preparations.
3 **Patches and gels**: Another way of delivering hormones is through the skin. This has the advantage of bypassing the digestive system but the disadvantage that people differ in the rate at which they absorb drugs this way. There can also be problems with reactions to the adhesive that keeps the patch applied.
4 **Implants**: Inserted under the skin an implant releases oestrogen slowly and needs to be replaced every four to 12 months, depending on the strength of implant used. Only oestrogen is available as an implant but it can be used in combination with progestogen tablets for women who still have their uterus and therefore need combina-tion treatment.
5 **Nasal spray**: Drugs can be well absorbed from the lining of the nose and one type of oestrogen treatment is available as a spray that's sniffed once daily (Aerodiol®).

Figure 2: Mirena ® intra-uterine system

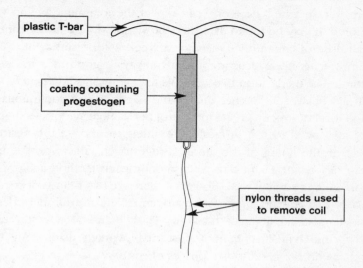

plastic T-bar

coating containing
progestogen

nylon threads used
to remove coil

Another option is an Intra-uterine system. Mirena® is exactly the same as a contraceptive 'coil' (intra-uterine device) in appearance except the shaft of the device is covered with a progestogen that's very slowly released into the cavity of the womb (see figure 2). Mirena® can take the place of progestogen tablets or patches used in other types of combined HRT, although strictly speaking this is as yet an 'unlicensed' use of the device in the UK.

Local treatments

Vaginal creams, pessaries and rings are intended to relieve the problems caused by the thinning and dryness of the vagina post-menopause. Creams and pessaries are usually applied once daily (evening time is often the most convenient), using the applicator device supplied. Vaginal rings last for three months before needing to be renewed. A course of local treatment for a few weeks may be enough to build up the vaginal lining sufficiently to relieve symptoms for some months thereafter, in which case one can repeat the treatment as and when required. It may be found that once the symptoms are under control a small dose of cream once or twice a week will be sufficient to keep the problems from recurring and it's always a good idea to use the minimum of medication that controls the symptoms adequately.

If a woman still has her uterus and needs to use continuous (i.e. daily) local oestrogen cream to control her vaginal symptoms then she may also need to use progestogen tablets to oppose the oestrogen effect on the lining of the uterus. Progestogen tablets can be taken every day or for 12–14 days each month; each method achieves the desired effect equally well. However, there are two brands of cream or pessary that contain a type of oestrogen called oestriol that does *not* over-stimulate the lining of the uterus. These brands are Ovestin® cream and Ortho-Gynest® cream or pessaries. Women using only these products do not need to use progestogens as well.

If a woman is using one of the other non-oestriol brands (Premarin® cream, Tampovagan® or Vagifem® pessaries) no more often than twice a week then there may not be a definite need to also use progestogen tablets because the total amount of oestrogen being used is small. There is also a feeling that the amount of oestrogen absorbed from the vaginal ring preparation (Estring®) is so low that additional progestogen is unnecessary. This decision should, however, be made on an individual basis after discussing it with your doctor.

The amount of oestrogen that's absorbed from the vagina and so travels to the rest of the body is quite small when using these products but some women do notice a decrease in flushes and sweats even if they are using a vaginal cream and nothing else. However, oestriol is a very weak oestrogen and only relieves vaginal symptoms, so women using Ovestin® or Ortho-Gynest® do not get general symptom relief from these products. As a general rule when using local treatments alone it is recommended that every few months one takes a break for a while to see if they are still needed.

Oral treatments

These are the commonest forms of HRT in regular use and are suitable for treating all types of menopausal symptoms. Oestrogen-only tablets (for women who've had their uterus removed) contain the same dose of oestrogen in every tablet. Examples include Climaval® and Hormonin®.

For combined oestrogen–progestogen preparations the situation is a little more complicated as there are two general groups in use:

1 **Sequential**: These attempt to mimic the natural monthly swing of the hormones in the pre-menopausal woman by providing a daily dose of oestrogen only for the first two weeks and then adding the progestogen in the second two weeks of each 28-day cycle. Sequential HRT preparations are used in women who wish to take HRT but who are in the climacteric, i.e. they are still getting natural periods (even if their cycle has become erratic). Because the level of progestogen goes up and down this type of HRT causes a monthly bleed, although mostly this is quite light. (See below for details of two variations on the sequential types of HRT.) Examples of sequential HRT are Elleste Duet® and Prempak-C®.

2 **Continuous**: These have the same dose of oestrogen and pro-gestogen in each tablet. The idea here is that by keeping the hormone levels steady no monthly bleeding will occur. Often in the first four to six months of using continuous HRT irregular bleeding does occur, but then settles down and disappears. Continuous HRT is mainly intended for use in women who have had no natural period for at least a year beforehand. Examples include Kliofem® and Nuvelle Continuous®.

There are dozens of available brands of HRT of all types, and a full list is on the NetDoctor website at www.netdoctor.co.uk/medicines. The main side effects of HRT are summarised in appendix B. (Incidentally one of the many bizarre rules that govern NHS prescription charges is that because sequential HRT brands contain a combination of two packs of drugs they cost two prescription charges, whereas continuous HRT costs only one.)

Variations on sequential HRT

INTERMITTENT

In one brand of sequential HRT (Cyclo-progynova®) oestrogen is taken for the first 11 days, then oestrogen + progestogen for 10 days and then there are seven days without treatment in each 28-day cycle. Usually there will be a light period in the pill-free week. This is an old type of HRT and is rarely used now.

LONG CYCLE

There must be very few women who regret leaving behind the chore of monthly periods, so for a post-menopausal woman to get periods back with HRT is not a big plus point. One of the great aims of HRT development over the years has been to achieve 'no bleed' treatment. This is one of the reasons why continuous HRT has come along. Generally speaking continuous HRT is successful in avoiding bleeding but most continuous HRT brands are intended for use only in women who are a year past their last period. Women who are still having some periods are usually given sequential HRT, which continues the monthly bleeding cycle. One brand gets round this problem a bit by going for a three-monthly cycle instead, so that the bleeds occur correspondingly less often. In this brand (Tridestra®) the oestrogen is given for 70 days in a row, then the progestogen is taken for 14 days. Seven dummy tablets (i.e. containing no active hormones) are then taken to give a gap before the next three-month sequence starts.

One of the issues about the safety of HRT concerns the relative merits of using sequential versus continuous combined HRT, but we'll come back to this in the next chapter and in the meantime continue with describing the various forms of HRT in use.

Patches and gels

PATCHES

Modern HRT patches are very thin, clear ovals or squares, which contain hormones within the adhesive layer. The hormones pass through the skin directly into the bloodstream and are distributed to the rest of the body. Many people like the convenience of patches, which can be changed every three to four days or seven days depending on the brand. Both oestrogen and progestogens can be given in this way and combinations of patches and tablets are also common. Every possible variation is available, from brands that use an oestrogen patch every 3 or 4 days and add progestogen tablets in the second half of each month to those that use entirely patches to provide continuous combined, sequential combined or oestrogen-only HRT.

Patches need to be applied to smooth skin below the waist and the adhesive is designed to withstand showering, etc. Changing the site of the patch helps avoid skin irritation, which is one of the practical problems that stops patches from working for some people.

GELS

Gels that provide a measured amount of oestrogen and are rapidly absorbed from the skin are popular and have the advantage of avoiding the irritation of patch adhesive. It's also possible to fine tune the amount of gel to use the minimum amount that controls symptoms. Such fine control is not so easily obtained with patches and tablets.

Implants

These take the form of a small pellet inserted under the skin, which releases oestrogen slowly over some months. The obvious advantage is that there's no need to remember to take tablets or change patches. The amount of oestrogen released is initially high and then drops off slowly and replacement of the implant needs to be done when the amount of oestrogen being released is insufficient for symptom control. When that is depends mostly on the starting dose, which is why there is such a wide range (about three to four months for the minimum dose pellets and 12 to 18 months for the highest dose). Women who have their uterus still need to take progesterone so they don't get away without taking tablets but in practice oestrogen implants are most often used in women who have had a hysterectomy (removal of the uterus).

The technique of inserting the implant is not difficult but is not one that is commonly done by GPs. Usually implants are done by a gynaecologist or a specialist at a menopause clinic, who are more used to judging the correct dose and timing of replacements. One other disadvantage of implants relates to the fact that high oestrogen levels can also cause sweats and flushes as easily as low levels. Therefore, some women paradoxically can be just as badly off if their dose is too high. The solution if that happens is to wait until the oestrogen level falls sufficiently, but that can mean a wait of several months.

Nasal spray

The oestrogen nasal spray does not have any particular advantages except perhaps in allowing fine dosage adjustment in the same way as a gel.

One of the points to note about using the minimum amount of HRT, of any type, that just controls symptoms is that such doses may not be enough to confer longer-term benefits such as protection against osteoporosis (chapter 7).

Intra-uterine system

The Mirena® intra-uterine system is a way of delivering progestogen directly to where it is needed; the lining of the uterus. Progestogen in tablets or patches travels everywhere in the body as well as to the uterus. Progestogens are thought to be more commonly responsible than oestrogens for many of the side effects of HRT such as headaches, bloating, mood swings and spotty skin.

The tiny amount of progestogen in Mirena® protects the lining of the womb from the excess effects of oestrogen without causing general side effects. Mirena® can also be very successful at cutting the menstrual flow in women with heavy periods and is an effective contraceptive device, so it has a number of useful properties. A Mirena® will need to be replaced every five years.

Other medicines used in the menopause

Other than oestrogen–progestogen hormone replacement and the complementary treatments that were covered in the last chapter there are several other treatments useful in the menopause. First the list, and then we'll go through them in detail:

- *Tibolone*: This is a unique type of HRT.
- *Alternatives to HRT*: These are conventional medicines offering menopausal symptom relief. Presently the main drug in this group is clonidine, which can give some relief from flushes. There are also non-hormonal vaginal treatments that can relieve vaginal dryness.
- *Treatments for irregular or heavy bleeding*: A common problem in the lead-up to the menopause.

- *Testosterone*: The 'male' hormone but it can have a role in treating loss of libido.
- *Treatments for osteoporosis*: Covered in detail in chapter 7.

Tibolone (Livial®)

Tibolone (brand name = Livial®) is a synthetic steroid hormone, taken in tablet form, which has some oestrogen *plus* some progesterone effects (and, in fact, also has some testosterone-like effects too). In a way it's a type of combined continuous HRT in a single tablet, which is largely how it's used. It helps flushes and sweats, vaginal dryness and irritation and also protects against osteoporosis. It possibly improves libido. It does not appear to be associated with some of the problems of conventional HRT that we'll be looking at in the next chapter. The benefits of tibolone include much less breast tenderness and no effect on breast tissue density in mammograms. It is therefore considered the most 'breast friendly' HRT.

Tibolone is only suitable for women who are post-menopause. If started in the pre-menopause phase there is a high chance it will cause irregular vaginal bleeding. In fact in the first few months of using it post-menopause this often occurs too, but settles down. It is likely that tibolone will become increasingly popular in view of its favourable balance of benefits versus side effects.

Alternatives to HRT

HRT is not suitable for all women for a variety of reasons. These include unacceptable side effects, a dislike for the return or the persistence of regular vaginal bleeding or concern over risks such as breast cancer, endometrial cancer or the development of clots in the veins. Other medicines exist that also give relief of menopausal symptoms to a greater or lesser degree.

CLONIDINE

Clonidine is a drug mainly used for the reduction of high blood pressure but at smaller doses it can help flushes. It has several side effects that can limit its use, including dry mouth, sedation and dizziness. Tolerance usually develops, so its effect wears off, but it can help initially.

VAGINAL TREATMENTS

Non-hormonal vaginal moisturisers and lubricants include Replens® and Senselle®. Neither of these is available on NHS prescription so they need to be purchased directly from a pharmacy.

Irregular or heavy vaginal bleeding

One of the common problems of the climacteric is that periods become erratic both in spacing and amount. Ultimately of course the periods peter out altogether but until that happens there can be plenty of problems from heavy bleeding as well. The problem is certainly not limited to the time around the menopause and about 5 per cent of women aged 30–49 consult their GP each year with heavy menstrual bleeding. It is the commonest reason for a woman to have her uterus removed (hysterectomy) – one in five women have had this done before the age of sixty.

MEDICAL TREATMENTS

Non-steroidal anti-inflammatory drugs (NSAIDs) are medicines like ibuprofen that are very commonly used as painkillers and to lower a raised temperature. They reduce the amount of blood lost in a period and help reduce pain. Mefenamic acid is another painkiller commonly used in the same way.

Tranexamic acid is a drug that encourages blood to clot on a bleeding surface and it can reduce heavy menstrual bleeding effectively. It's used just for the heaviest three or four days of each period. It's not suitable for women with a previous history of clots in the veins (thrombosis). Nausea, vomiting and diarrhoea are the likeliest side effects from this drug.

Oral progestogen tablets given for long enough (21 days each cycle) will cut menstrual flow, as will the progestogen released from the Mirena® intra-uterine system. Mirena® is currently the most effective medical (i.e. non-surgical) way of dealing with excessive vaginal bleeding.

There are other drug options that can be used by specialists if necessary but these can be accompanied by significant side effects.

SURGICAL TREATMENTS

Complete removal of the uterus is a relatively major operation and therefore is accompanied by risks such as those of an anaesthetic, bleeding at operation, wound infection, vein clots post-operatively and so on. These are risks that apply to any such operation and in practice hysterectomy is a successful and well-tolerated procedure. Lesser procedures are now possible using fibre-optic instruments that can destroy the lining of the uterus (endometrial ablation). This works because it is only the inner lining of the uterus that is hormone-sensitive and responsible for menstruation.

The procedure does not completely remove every single piece of the uterine lining, and 30–90 per cent of women still get some menstrual bleeding afterwards, but usually it is light. For the same reason a woman who has endometrial ablation and who later takes HRT will still need to use a combined HRT preparation and not just oestrogen alone.

Testosterone

The distinction between 'female hormones' and 'male hormones' is to some extent artificial. Both men and women naturally produce oestrogen, progesterone and testosterone. Prior to the menopause women produce less than a tenth of the amount of testosterone found in men, but after the menopause this amount slowly increases. The ovaries are the main source of testosterone in women but it is also made in fatty tissue, so being overweight is an extra factor that can push testosterone levels up.

Excess testosterone in women encourages greasy skin and the growth of facial hair. It can also increase the risk of heart attack and stroke in women who are at greater risk for these problems. This might apply, for example, to a woman with high blood pressure, high cholesterol in the blood, a family history of heart disease or stroke or who smoked.

Having said all that, one might therefore wonder why testosterone can be a treatment option for menopausal women. The reason is that it appears to boost energy levels and libido, although not in everyone. A drop in libido is so common at the time of the menopause it could be considered normal, but that doesn't mean it can't be a problem. Sexual interest affects and is affected by relationships so one needs to be careful that libido problems are not just blamed on hormone lack. As with the menopause in general, that can be too simple an explanation and the source of much disappointment if HRT does not 'fix' it easily.

Women who have had their ovaries removed before the menopause often experience a major loss of libido and the role of testosterone replacement for them is now well established. For women going through the natural menopause the exact role of testosterone replacement is much less clear. Unfortunately there is no blood test that can show if testosterone treatment will help: it is a case of trial and error.

USING TESTOSTERONE TREATMENT

The method used at some Menopause Clinics to determine if testosterone replacement will be helpful involves the daily use of the male testosterone patch (Andropatch® 2.5mg) over a period of 2–4 weeks. These patches cannot be used for longer than this in women as they give too high a level of testosterone but during the trial period it should be possible for a woman to judge if it's having a positive effect on her libido. If so then she can consider having a testosterone implant inserted. (Testosterone patches specifically designed for women are being developed but are not yet available.)

Like oestrogen implants, testosterone implants are small pellets that are inserted under the skin. A testosterone implant dissolves slowly over 6–8 months and cannot be removed easily once it's inserted, so if side effects develop then you've got to wait until they wear off. Testosterone implants are not recommended in the higher-risk women noted above and they should always be combined with HRT in some form after the menopause. If achieving the desired effect they can be replaced every 6–8 months.

Key Points

- Hormone replacement therapy (HRT) comprises either oestrogen alone or oestrogen combined with a progestogen.
- Women who still have their uterus always need the combined type of HRT, containing both oestrogen and progestogen.
- Combined HRT is of two types: sequential (in which the hormone dose varies through the month) and continuous (in which the hormone levels are steady). Continuous oestrogen-only treatments always have a steady dose.
- If menopausal symptoms are localised only to the vagina and bladder area then local oestrogen creams may suffice.

- Heavy menstrual bleeding can be treated by hormones, a progestogen-releasing intra-uterine system, removal of the uterine lining or hysterectomy.
- Testosterone treatment may have a role in treating reduced libido at the menopause.

Chapter 6

The Pros and Cons of Hormone Replacement Therapy

There is no doubt that HRT is an important and useful treatment but it's also true that there has been a shake-up of opinion over its pros and cons in the very recent past.

If we go back just a couple of years the accepted wisdom was that on top of menopausal symptom relief HRT gave major health benefits including reductions in coronary heart disease (heart attacks), osteoporosis (weakening of the bones) and cancer of the bowel. On the down side HRT increased the risk for developing breast cancer and vein thrombosis. Many critics, however, felt that the benefits of HRT were possibly exaggerated or artificial because women who sought and were receiving HRT were more likely to be generally health conscious. Thus they would in any case be less likely to get heart disease, osteoporosis and bowel cancer because they took better care of themselves than women who did not seek or receive HRT. Whatever the accuracy of those assumptions the result was that there were too many question marks over HRT and more research was needed.

Several large research studies were set up, principally in the USA and the UK, to provide the answers. The results of the American studies came through first, and have put the cat among the pigeons. It's worth knowing some of the details of these studies to understand the context of what was discovered and the relevance it's had to HRT knowledge.

Heart and Estrogen Replacement Study (HERS)

This study was designed to see if HRT affected heart disease. Over two and a half thousand American women, with an average age of 67 years, and who were already known to have heart disease were entered. These women had a history of a heart attack or had medical investigations that proved they had narrowing of the heart's own blood vessels, which is what is meant by the term 'coronary heart disease'. The form of HRT used was a combination of conjugated oestrogens and a progestogen called medroxyprogesterone. This combination is the most commonly used in the USA and is similar to the brand available in the UK called Premique®, except that the dose of medroxyprogesterone in Premique® is twice that used in the HERS study.

Medical studies like this are organised so that half of the subjects receive the active treatment (HRT) and the other half receive a dummy (placebo) treatment. Not until the end of the study do the patients or the doctors know who received what, which increases the accuracy of the observations made.

The initial study ran for just over four years but because many women remained under observation it was possible to complete a second report, called 'HERS II' that looked at the data collected over nearly seven years. It was the HERS II results, published in July 2002, that caused the first stir because contrary to earlier expectations HRT had no benefit on the outcome for heart disease. Women on HRT were just as likely as those who were not to have a further heart attack or to die from heart disease.

Other results from the HERS II were also unfavourable. They showed that the women on HRT had about twice the chance of having a vein thrombosis during the entire period of study and that this risk was highest in the first couple of years of using HRT. Gallbladder problems such as gallstones were also more common in the women on HRT.

These results went against one of the major assumptions of HRT up to that point in time, which was that it was helpful in coronary heart disease. Two weeks later the results of another, much larger study (the Women's Health Initiative) were published that really rocked the foundations underpinning the use of HRT.

Women's Health Initiative Study (WHI)

This was another large American study, this time involving over sixteen thousand women who were post-menopausal and in the age range 50–79. It used the same form of HRT as the HERS study (conjugated oestrogens + medroxyprogesterone) and looked at the effects HRT had on coronary heart disease, breast cancer and a number of other conditions such as stroke, thrombosis and bowel cancer. As with the HERS trial this one used a group taking treatment and another taking placebo.

The trial was planned to last 8.5 years but was stopped early at 5.2 years because of an increase in the number of women on HRT who were developing breast cancer. Increases were also seen in coronary heart disease, stroke and vein thrombosis. However, there were reductions in hip fracture and colon cancer and overall there was no effect on death rates between the two groups. The impact of the

WHI study, which was much larger in size and scope than the HERS study, has been considerable around the world.

WISDOM Study

The women's international study of long duration oestrogen after menopause (WISDOM) is a UK based study, started by the Medical Research Council (MRC) in 1999, that was designed to look at many of the same issues as the WHI study and it was due to run until 2016. The WHI results, however, caused the MRC to abandon most of the WISDOM trial in November 2002. One section of the WISDOM trial, looking at the effects of oestrogen alone on women who have had a hysterectomy, is still ongoing.

Risks in perspective

HRT does not directly cause heart disease, strokes, breast cancer or vein thrombosis. These are all conditions that occur in women who don't take HRT and there are many other factors that can increase a woman's risk that are unrelated to hormones, such as her family history, smoking history, blood pressure and cholesterol level to mention only a few. We don't know precisely why these risk factors matter, but the more that are present the more likely it is that the chain of events that leads to these health problems will be set in motion.

To put into perspective the magnitude of the risks of HRT it helps to put together some figures. To aid comparison the risks are stated as the number of people affected per 10,000 women-years of observation (e.g. 5,000 women observed over two years = 10,000 women-years. 1,000 women observed over 10 years is also 10,000 women years).

HEART DISEASE

The WHI study showed that women not taking HRT (i.e. on placebo) had 30 cases of heart disease per 10,000 women-years, whereas on HRT it was 37 per 10,000 women-years.

STROKE

On placebo the risk was 21 per 10,000 women-years. On HRT the risk was 29 per 10,000 women-years.

CLOTS IN THE VEINS (VENOUS THROMBOSIS)

(Researchers included those clots that moved from the leg veins up into the lungs, which are the most dangerous type, as well as those that stayed within the leg veins. The condition in which clots travel to the lungs is called pulmonary embolism.)

On placebo the risk was 16 per 10,000 women-years. On HRT the risk was 34 per 10,000 women-years.

ENDOMETRIAL CANCER (CANCER OF THE LINING OF THE WOMB)

It is difficult to put an exact figure on it but long-term HRT does increase the risk of endometrial cancer. Using combined HRT reduces the risk of this happening, but does not eliminate it. There is some evidence to suggest that sequential HRT (which is the sort associated with a monthly bleed and is the recommended type for women in the pre-menopause or climacteric phase) is associated eventually with a slightly higher risk than continuous HRT. Ideally, therefore, all women on long-term HRT should move to a continuous type within a year or two of starting HRT if they can.

Breast disease and HRT

There are several important issues to cover concerning breast disease and HRT.

BREAST CANCER

In the WHI study the risk of developing breast cancer on placebo was 30 per 10,000 women-years and on HRT the risk was 38 per 10,000 women-years. HRT has been known for years to increase the risk of breast cancer. The risk increases with the length of time that HRT is used and becomes detectable after about five years of treatment. The risk falls once HRT is stopped, and takes about five years to drop back to the average in the population.

Stating the breast cancer risk another way to illustrate this, in women aged 50 who do not use HRT about 45 in every thousand will be diagnosed with breast cancer by the time they reach the age of 70. In women who start HRT at age 50 and use it for five years the figure would be 47 in every thousand. In those who take HRT for 10 years breast cancer will occur in 51 in a thousand and for 15 years it will be 57 in a thousand.

The best presently available evidence tells us that breast cancers that occur in women taking HRT are smaller, less advanced and of a more treatable type than breast cancers occurring in women not taking HRT. This accounts for the fact that despite the increased numbers of cancers arising due to HRT, the actual mortality of women from breast cancer is the same in the HRT and non-HRT populations. Some breast cancer experts feel, however, that the balance of risk has swung against HRT given for longer than five years. As is made clear next, there are additional factors to consider.

OTHER BREAST PROBLEMS RELATED TO HRT

Women in the pre-menopause who take HRT often get breast pain and benign breast lumps, including cysts (fluid-filled lumps). HRT may cause benign breast lumps that are already present to get bigger. In the UK we place great emphasis not only on the need for a woman to check her breasts regularly and report any changes to her doctor but also we have a national screening service that offers periodic mammograms to women over 50. HRT is known to increase the density of breast tissue, which makes it harder for the X-rays used in mammography to penetrate the breast. It is therefore of concern that HRT can make it more difficult to detect breast cancer by mammography.

Unanswered questions

The results of these studies have raised as many questions as they have answered. Perhaps even more so as the WHI and WISDOM trials were closed before they could resolve many of the original issues that they were hoped to clarify. In particular we don't know for sure if the results found in these studies, which used a particular type of HRT (conjugated oestrogens and medroxyprogesterone) are applicable to all the other types of HRT. There are subtle differences between the various oestrogens and progestogens in use and it is unknown if they have different risks attached – they might be better or worse. In the meantime we have to generalise and say that the results from the WHI and HERS studies should be applied to all types of combined HRT. It may be that it is now too difficult to set up yet more studies to get answers to all the questions the experts feel are still uncertain. We'll therefore need to say that what we now know is as much as we are going to know for some years yet, and that is the basis upon which decisions on HRT have to be made.

The benefits of HRT

Taking all the most recent information into account and bearing in mind that not all of these are experienced by every woman, we can restate the benefits of HRT thus:

- improved general sense of well-being,
- diminished hot flushes and night sweats,
- less fatigue,
- improved mood,
- relief from vaginal dryness and urinary symptoms,
- protection against the development of osteoporosis,
- possible protection against bowel cancer.

The disadvantages of HRT

MINOR (MAINLY SHORT-TERM AND IMPROVE WITH TIME OR ADJUSTMENT OF THE HRT)
- vaginal bleeding which may be heavy, painful or irregular,
- fluid retention (but weight gain has *not* been shown to be a definite side effect of HRT),
- breast tenderness,
- increased risk of developing benign breast lumps.

MAJOR (MAINLY ARISE FROM LONG-TERM TREATMENT)
- increased risk of breast cancer (and practical problems in mammography screening),
- increased risk of vein thrombosis and pulmonary embolism (especially in the first 12 to 18 months of treatment),
- possible increased risk of heart disease and stroke in older women (especially in the first 12 to 18 months of treatment),
- increased risk of endometrial cancer.

There is a lot of information in this chapter and it's not very easy to take in. Many doctors too find it difficult to be sure of the right advice to give a woman concerning the menopause, particularly in respect of HRT. Now, more than ever, decisions on menopause treatment need to be tailored to the needs and the circumstances of the individual woman. It is possible to make sense of it all though, and chapter 8 tries to provide some signposts to guide you through the maze.

Before going that far we need to look at one of the major issues concerning women after the menopause (and older men too): osteoporosis.

Key Points

- The results of recent research studies have altered our understanding of the risks and benefits of HRT, or more exactly of combined HRT.
- These studies showed that HRT does not protect a woman with coronary heart disease from further development of this problem and that HRT increases the risks of getting vein clots, gall bladder disease, stroke, breast cancer and endometrial cancer.
- The heart and vein risks are most pronounced in the first 18 months on HRT, whereas the effect on the breasts and uterus may take five years or more to develop.
- It is uncertain if the problems revealed in these studies are applicable to all types of combined HRT, but we have to assume this is so for now.
- HRT effectively relieves the symptoms of the menopause, protects against osteoporosis and probably lowers a woman's risk of getting bowel cancer.
- Experts are now less likely to recommend using combined HRT for longer than five years, but this may still be appropriate for an individual woman once all her circumstances are considered.

Chapter 7

Osteoporosis

Osteoporosis is the condition in which the amount of bone in the body is reduced below what is normal for a person's sex and age. Put simply, osteoporosis causes weaker bones, and thus increases the likelihood of breaking a bone.

Bone structure

Bone has a complex structure that achieves the maximum amount of strength for the least amount of weight. It's a living tissue that can adapt according to circumstances to a certain extent. Thus it can increase its thickness in areas subjected to repeated heavy loads or repair itself when broken. Bone is also the site of manufacture of most of the components of blood (the bone marrow).

A typical bone such as the femur (upper leg bone) in cross section has an outer shell of very hard bone while in the middle space it has a honeycomb structure, through which is mingled the bone marrow (figure 3). Bone is made up mostly of protein fibres called collagen, upon which are laid down crystals made from calcium and phosphate that give bone its ability to withstand compression and bending forces. If you take a piece of bone and chemically leach these minerals out it becomes flexible and rubbery.

Under the microscope one sees that scattered throughout bone are two types of specialised cells. One type continually makes new bone (these are called 'osteoblasts') and the other group continuously dissolve bone into its component materials (the 'osteoclasts'). Bone is always on the go and the actions of bone manufacture and disassembly are usually almost exactly balanced. When increased loads are repeatedly put upon a bone then the osteoblasts become more active, thus laying down more bone locally and increasing the strength of this region. When a bone is fractured, osteoblasts go into overdrive around the fracture site and lay down more collagen fibres, then minerals on top to strengthen them. On average about 10 per cent of the skeleton is 're-modelled' annually, so in effect we get a new skeleton every ten years!

Aging and bone strength

It is normal for bone to get a bit weaker each year after the age of about 35, when our bones are at their maximum strength. Men tend to have greater bone mass than women of the same age but from this age both sexes lose about 1 per cent of their bone mass every year. Oestrogen stimulates the bone-forming cells, so when oestrogen levels drop after the menopause women have an increased rate of bone loss for between three and ten years thereafter. Then their rate of bone loss slows up to equal that of men, by which time a woman may have fallen considerably below the bone mass of a man the same age.

Figure 3: Normal and osteoporotic bone structures

NORMAL BONE

bone surface →

internal
meshwork of
bone →

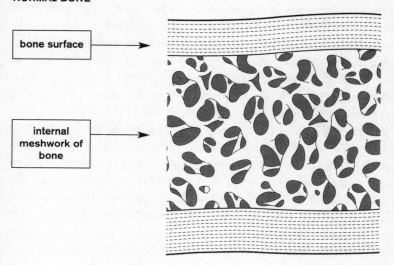

OSTEOPOROTIC BONE

thinner, weaker
lattice of bone →

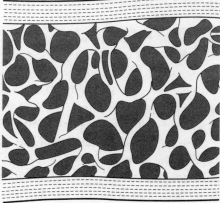

Defining osteoporosis

Defining when bones are abnormally weak has to take account of what is normal for the two sexes and the different age groups. Ultimately osteoporotic bone is at higher risk than average of breaking, but waiting for that to happen or only defining osteoporotic bones as broken ones is hardly satisfactory; what we need to do is measure bone strength before it breaks, so that extra corrective action can be taken in advance for those people at high risk.

Devices to measure the density of bones are now available and have allowed researchers to build up information on bone strength across the population. By comparing an individual's readings against a reference standard (the average bone strength of young adults) one can say whether a person's bones are normal strength, slightly weaker (the correct term is 'osteopenia') or very weak (osteoporosis).

For those who like to know the details and understand mathematics osteoporosis is defined as a bone density more than 2.5 standard deviations below the mean for young adults. The rest of us can just remember that this is called the 'T score' and that osteoporosis exists if the T score is less than −2.5.

Types of fracture in osteoporosis

As osteoporotic bones are weak they may fracture too easily, i.e. in circumstances that would not break a normal bone. These are called 'low impact' or 'osteoporotic' fractures. Fractures in bone affected by osteoporosis are also most likely in areas where there is a greater percentage of the honeycomb type of bone, which is less able to take the shock of a fall. These are the forearm (especially the wrist), the femur close to the hip joint (called the 'neck' of the femur) and the vertebrae of the spine.

A low impact fracture is one that occurs from a fall from standing height or less and fractures of the hip, wrist or forearm can be categorised in this way fairly easily. It is more difficult to do so for the spine as many spinal fractures occur out of the blue and are not related to falls – sometimes they are not even accompanied by much pain. However, the sudden onset of back pain should suggest there has been a collapsed vertebra, possibly due to osteoporosis. Medical investigations are usually necessary to check that a low impact fracture is definitely due to osteoporosis and not one of the many other diseases that can potentially weaken bones, but this is usually quite straight-forward for a doctor to do.

The scale of the problem

One in three women and 1 in 12 men over the age of 50 will suffer a fracture of the hip, wrist or spine as a result of osteoporosis, which in total causes 310,000 fractures in the UK annually. The estimated cost to the country of treating these fractures is enormous at £1.7 billion each year, but the cost to the individual can be higher than a sum of money:

- Bone fractures can cause considerable pain and disability.
- 50 per cent of people who suffer a fractured hip lose the ability to live independently.
- Around 20 per cent of elderly people who fracture a hip die within a year as a result of their fracture.

Detection of osteoporosis

The majority of people who suffer a fracture from osteoporosis are not known to have the condition prior to breaking their bone. Osteoporosis is an under-recognised condition, which is partly because in the UK we have not developed an organised approach to detecting it. As a result we do not yet consistently seek people at high risk of getting a fracture and offer them appropriate advice or treatment to reduce their risk. Many people who have had a fracture due to osteoporosis do not receive the follow-up treatment that helps reduce the chances of their getting another one.

There are wide variations between the different regions of the UK in the quality and quantity of effort put in to detecting and treating osteoporosis, and further divisions in the quality of care delivered to people from different social groups. For example, in a study carried out in Glasgow people from the most deprived areas were eight times less likely to be referred for the tests to detect osteoporosis than those from the most affluent areas.

There is, however, some good news too. The government has recognised the deficiencies that exist in osteoporosis management nationally and more funding is slowly coming through to expand the services, such as bone scanning machines to help diagnose it as well as specialists in osteoporosis. A 'Primary Care Strategy for Osteoporosis and Falls' was published in October 2002 that set out standards for osteoporosis care that ought to be achieved by Primary Care Organisations. As with all such initiatives the publication of a document, although important, won't achieve much without the other resources coming along to match but it does at least show what needs to be done.

Diagnosing osteoporosis

The best test to diagnose osteoporosis is a scan, which uses a very small dose of X-rays to measure the density of the bones. Usually the same reference point in the skeleton is chosen, which allows better comparison between different people. The hip, forearm, heel bone or spine are all used but exactly which varies according to local procedure. The technique is called a 'DEXA' scan – short for dual-energy X-ray absorpiometry. Ultrasound of the heel bone is another common technique and uses cheaper equipment but it's not yet clear if it's as accurate or reliable as DEXA scanning.

Ordinary X-rays are not reliable as a tool for diagnosing osteoporosis, for various technical reasons. It can be possible to *suspect* from a standard X-ray film that the person has less bone mass than normal as the bone outline on the film might appear fainter, but the same appearance will show if the exposure of the film is slightly too high. Conversely if the film is slightly underexposed then the bones will look normally dense. In any case as much as 30 per cent of bone mass needs to be lost before it shows up on ordinary X-rays. DEXA scanning is designed to get round these limitations.

Who needs a bone scan?

There are not yet enough of these DEXA scanners across the UK to make the test freely available to everyone who wants one, so some form of vetting procedure is used to try and ensure that those most at need of being scanned are tested. The details of these criteria vary a bit around the country but the following list is a representative guide (the presence of any one factor on this list is enough to justify a DEXA scan):

- A woman over 50 who has had a low impact fracture.
- Anyone taking oral steroid (prednisolone 5mg daily or greater for 3 or more months).
- A woman under 45 who has had an early menopause or removal of the ovaries but who has not received HRT up to the 'average' age at the menopause of about 50.
- A woman who is around the menopause who also has any two of the following:
  - She smokes.
  - She has a body mass index (BMI – see below) less than 21.
  - She has a history in her mother of a hip fracture below 80 years of age.
  - She drinks more than 35 units of alcohol weekly (see below).

- A man with a high alcohol consumption of over 50 units of alcohol weekly.

People who are unusually thin are more likely to develop osteoporosis, and the way to define 'thin-ness' is to measure the body mass index (BMI). The BMI relates a person's weight to their height and therefore can be applied to any person, whether tall or short, and to both sexes.

BODY MASS INDEX

Weight and height are related and knowledge of both is needed before one can say if a person is overweight, under weight or just right. A simple mathematical formula relating the two is now universally used to do this – the Body Mass Index (BMI). To calculate a BMI, take the person's weight (in kilograms) and divide it by the square of their height (in metres). For example an 80kg person of height 1.7m will have a BMI of $80/(1.7 \times 1.7) = 27.7 \, kg/m^2$ (the BMI formula applies equally to men and women). The ranges of BMI are:

- Normal   =   20–24.9
- Overweight =   25–30
- Obese   =   Over 30

People with a BMI of 21 or less have a higher rate of bone loss than those who are heavier, and obese people have lower rates of bone loss than those who are ideal weight. It is not known if a thin person who deliberately puts on a lot of weight will reduce their subsequent fracture risk. Obesity, of course, carries with it many other health hazards.

Causes of osteoporosis

Osteoporosis is not yet fully understood but we know quite a lot about what increases the risk of a person getting it and some things that can be done to prevent it. Osteoporosis basically occurs because of an increased rate of bone loss, and there are three groups of factors that influence this:

1 those that you can do nothing about,
2 those that are under your own control,
3 causes related to other medical conditions or drug therapy.

1. UNCHANGEABLE CAUSES OF INCREASED BONE LOSS
- increasing age
- family history of osteoporosis
- female sex
- following natural menopause
- being thin (although putting on weight again may cancel the bone loss).

2. CHANGEABLE CAUSES OF INCREASED BONE LOSS
- inactivity
- poor diet (low in calcium)
- smoking
- increased alcohol intake (see below).

3. MEDICALLY-RELATED CAUSES OF INCREASED BONE LOSS
- steroid drug treatment (especially if prolonged more than a few weeks)
- early menopause or the removal of the ovaries at a young age (under 45 years) not followed by HRT

- hormone abnormalities (such as over-activity of the thyroid gland, or of the glands which produce the body's natural steroids, or under-production of testosterone in men).

ALCOHOL

High levels of alcohol intake (over 50 units per week in men, or 35 units in women) are associated with osteoporosis. It is possible that lower levels of alcohol consumption than this could still damage bone, and we know that you don't need to drink this heavily to be at higher risk of a whole range of other medical problems caused by alcohol.

Prevention and treatment of osteoporosis

GENERAL MEASURES

It's unlikely that we could abolish osteoporosis but ideally it could be prevented from occurring in a high proportion of people who are currently at risk. Given our present state of knowledge and ability to influence it however, it will be some time before we make a big impact on the problem. It should, however, be obvious from the above that healthy bones at least partially reflect healthy living. Taking regular exercise is the single most important action anyone can take to improve the strength of their bones. Exercise also greatly reduces the risk of heart disease, high blood pressure and diabetes and it has positive effects on mental well-being too. The sort of exercise that is beneficial is weight-bearing, such as walking or aerobics. *Excessive* running may, however, cause increased bone loss and as some running enthusiasts are also very thin they should take advice on the best way to avoid bone problems later in life. The majority of us who are not in the elite athlete category need not be so concerned. Stopping smoking also reduces the chance of developing osteoporosis.

DIET

A good calcium intake is essential throughout life for healthy bones and there is good evidence that the adequacy of a child's diet at least partially determines their osteoporosis risk in adulthood. Although dairy products are high in calcium they are not the only source. Non-dairy food sources include:

- nuts and pulses (almonds, Brazil nuts, hazelnuts, sesame seeds),
- green leafy vegetables (broccoli, spinach, watercress, curly kale),
- dried fruits (apricots, dates, figs),
- fish (mackerel, pilchards, salmon, sardines),
- tofu and various calcium-fortified foods.

The daily intake of calcium required by an adult is around 800 milligrams. On average 250ml or half a pint of cow's milk or 150g/5oz of yoghurt contains 300 milligrams of calcium and low-fat dairy products contain the same amount of calcium as higher fat varieties. Calcium supplements can be bought and there are several types available on prescription if someone's dietary intake is low or marginal. Frail, elderly people with poor mobility may be helped by taking a supplement of calcium along with vitamin D. This type of supplement is safe but is best discussed with a doctor first.

These general measures can be used by everyone, whether or not they ultimately are shown to have osteoporosis. More detailed intervention depends on individual circumstances and so only an overview can be presented here. There are several types of treatment available, and often a combination will be more appropriate than just one.

HORMONE REPLACEMENT THERAPY

HRT slows the rate at which bone is lost after the menopause and may even reverse the process of osteoporosis, at least temporarily. The degree of protection from osteoporosis that HRT provides depends to a large extent on how long the HRT is used and until recently a period of 10 years' treatment was suggested as the optimum length of time for maximum bone protection while minimising the risks of HRT. The results of studies such as the Women's Health Initiative have cast doubt on such recommendations. The fact is that we do not presently know the best compromise between using HRT for bone protection versus the risks of using HRT. At present, however, most experts would suggest HRT up to about the age of 55 would be appropriate for a woman at high risk of developing osteoporosis.

SELECTIVE ESTROGEN RECEPTOR MODULATOR (SERM)

This is a fairly new type of drug, of which raloxifene (Evista) is presently the only available one. Raloxifene stimulates bone growth just as oestrogens do but has an anti-oestrogen effect on the uterus (womb) and on breast tissue. The latter effect is seen as desirable as it may reduce the tendency for long-term oestrogen-based HRT to increase the risk of developing breast cancer. Like oestrogen, raloxifene may, however, increase the risk of developing blood clots in the veins and cannot be used by a woman with a past history of deep vein thrombosis. It is preferably used only in women who are at least one year past their menopause and would be an option for a woman between about 55 and 70 years of age. Raloxifene has been shown to reduce the occurrence of spinal fractures, but not hip fractures.

BISPHOSPHONATES

This is a group of drugs that slows the rate at which bone is dissolved, thus favouring a build-up in bone strength over time. Several types are in common use and more are in the pipeline. Alendronate (Fosamax®) and risendronate (Actonel®) are the drugs of choice as they have the best evidence to show they reduce the rates of fracture in the spine and the hip. The incidence of spine, hip and forearm fractures may fall by as much as 50 per cent with alendronate in post-menopausal women with confirmed osteoporosis. Etidronate (Didronel PMO®) was the first available bisphosphonate and is still in widespread use but although it can reduce the rate of occurrence of vertebral fractures there is no evidence that it reduces fracture risk elsewhere.

All of the bisphosphonates can cause digestive side effects, particularly irritation of the gullet, which can limit their use in many people. This can be minimised by taking measures such as swallowing them down with plenty of water and avoiding lying down for at least half an hour after taking them. Other side effects are given in appendix B.

OTHER TREATMENTS

These are quite specialised and not commonly used. Calcitonin is a hormone given by injection but it is less effective than HRT or the bisphosphonates and has a number of potential side effects, including allergic reactions. Calcitriol is a vitamin D-like compound that can be used in osteoporosis caused by steroid drugs.

Hip protectors are shock-absorbing pads that can be worn to cushion the impact over the hip bone should a person fall down. They spread the load across a wider area of the upper leg and are useful as an extra measure in an elderly person prone to falls. They come as a sort of girdle with padding at the sides but it can be difficult for patients to remember to always put it on, or to want to keep it on.

Compliance is the business of sticking to the prescribed treatment, whether it is tablets or protective clothing and as osteoporosis treatment and prevention needs to be taken for years poor compliance can be a major issue in treating the condition. Elderly people are the most at risk of falls, and are also the most likely to become muddled about pills or suffer more severe side effects from them. Those in sheltered or supervised environments can be given help to remember their medication but where this is not possible and someone is forgetful then using a once-weekly dose of bisphosphonate supervised by a carer or nurse might be more reliable than a daily dose that depends entirely on the patient.

It is possible to combine treatments such as HRT and a bisphosphonate for a woman who is at high risk of osteoporosis or who wishes to do everything possible to reduce her osteoporosis risk. However, studies have not been done to quantify the degree of extra bone protection that would arise from such combinations.

Osteoporosis and men

Women tend to get more coverage in osteoporosis than men as they live longer, have generally weaker bones and ultimately more of them have an osteoporotic fracture. Men do, however, also develop osteoporosis and show an increase in osteoporotic hip fractures after the age of about 70 similar that shown by women five to ten years younger. More detail on the 'male menopause' is in chapter 9.

Key Points

- Osteoporosis is the condition in which bone mass and strength are reduced from normal.
- Bone is an active tissue in which the processes of bone manufacture and removal are normally in balance.
- Bone strength naturally declines with age and is less in women than in men of the same age.
- The rate of bone loss accelerates for a few years in women following the menopause.
- Men also experience osteoporosis but have fewer fractures compared to women.
- Diagnosing osteoporosis is most accurately done by DEXA scans of bone density.

- Everyone can help to protect themselves against osteoporosis by adopting a healthy lifestyle and in particular by remaining as active as possible.
- Adequate dietary calcium intake should be ensured in everyone, if necessary with the addition of calcium supplements.
- The main specific treatments and preventive measures for osteoporosis include hormone replacement therapy and SERM treatment for women and bisphosphonate treatment for both sexes.
- People on long-term oral steroids should receive bone protection with bisphosphonates.

Chapter 8

Menopause Treatment – Making the right choice

Chapter 6, by necessity, had to cover a lot of the bad points concerning HRT. There are no completely safe choices in medicine, just as life itself is accompanied by some degree of risk. Minimising risks is achievable, but avoiding them completely is not. However, as we've hopefully made clear, HRT is only one of many available treatments for the menopause, and choosing the right treatment involves taking an overall look at what problems (if any) are being caused by the menopause and then deciding on the treatment options.

The following four questions may help point you to the right answer for yourself.

1. Is the menopause causing symptoms?

Back in chapter 1 (table 1) there was a list of symptoms possibly attributable to the menopause. Individually these are all common problems with multiple possible explanations, but the more that are going on at the same time in a woman of the appropriate age the more likely it is that the menopause is causing them. Initially it is the symptoms that matter, and for most women this is the main reason they take any treatment at all.

If a woman has no relevant symptoms then taking any form of treatment becomes much more an issue of choice rather than necessity, with the main exception being a woman at high risk of developing osteoporosis (see below).

If there is a case for treatment to control symptoms only, then a range of complementary as well as conventional treatments is available. As far as the latter is concerned one can choose either local treatment such as oestrogen cream or general HRT.

2. Are there specific situations that need attention?

EARLY MENOPAUSE
It's our present understanding that oestrogen is important to the well-being of a woman in her reproductive years and that the balancing effect of progesterone on the uterine lining is also necessary. Therefore, women who experience the menopause early (under the age of about 45 years) are exposed to several years less of these female hormones than the average, and this is probably not bene-ficial to them. Certainly they are at increased risk of developing osteoporosis, and probably other health disadvantages too. In such women the use of HRT, up until the age of about 50, is a replacement for the natural oestrogen (and progesterone) that would otherwise be there. In these circumstances the benefits of HRT generally outweigh the risks. Only conventional HRT will, however, confer

those benefits, as complementary treatments have not been shown to match HRT in this respect.

OSTEOPOROSIS

Hopefully the checklists in the previous chapter will make it clear whether you are personally at increased risk of getting osteoporosis. If so then please discuss this with your doctor, and find out how you stand about getting a DEXA bone scan done. If this confirms you are already low then you need to consider all of the treatments previously outlined, particularly the bisphosphonate drugs, but HRT too. If you are at high risk, because of your family history for example, but presently your bone density reading is normal then you can still take all the relevant lifestyle measures (diet, exercise, etc) and another scan in a year or two will show whether you are winning or losing. Women who know they will be taking a reasonably high dose of steroid drugs for more than a few weeks should seriously consider using a bisphosphonate right from the start as much of the bone loss from long-term steroids occurs early on.

CARDIOVASCULAR DISEASE

Until the WHI study came along women with a high risk of developing cardiovascular disease (angina or past history of a heart attack) would have been recommended to take HRT. This is no longer so as far as combined HRT (oestrogen plus progestogen) is concerned. The jury is still out on whether oestrogen alone may benefit women with raised cardiovascular risk.

Cardiovascular risk is contributed to by many other important factors in addition to hormone levels, including general lifestyle, presence of smoking and high blood pressure, etc. All of these issues need to be looked at and dealt with too.

BOWEL CANCER

HRT appears to slightly reduce the risk of getting bowel cancer in the general population. Although it is beyond the scope of this book to cover the issue adequately some people are at increased risk of developing bowel cancer. For women in this group it may therefore be an extra factor that is in favour of taking HRT. However, there are no studies that actually show HRT helps reduce the risk of getting bowel cancer in people who at higher risk of getting it.

ALZHEIMER'S DISEASE

Alzheimer's disease is the commonest reason for people to develop dementia as they get older. Among the many effects of dementia are memory loss, personality changes, difficulties in coping with daily living tasks, disorientation and impairment of reasoning.

Studies published just a few years ago suggested that taking HRT, especially for periods over a year, reduced the likelihood of a woman later developing Alzheimer's disease. Doubts have arisen over the accuracy of this concept, again as a result of the Women's Health Initiative study, which indicated an *increased* risk of dementia in women over 65 taking the combined HRT used in this study. We need to be careful about drawing conclusions from this result for several reasons. First is that the age group over 65 in the study is generally older than that in the UK of women regularly taking HRT. Second, we don't know if the particular oestrogen/progestogen combination used in the WHI study, which is not exactly the same as that available for prescription in the UK, is peculiar in some way that other combined HRT forms are not. Third, we don't know if the use of oestrogen-only HRT will be accompanied by the same results – this is one of the reasons that this part of the WHI and the WISDOM studies have been continued.

There is no evidence that HRT improves Alzheimer's disease once it has become established.

3. Are there any definite reasons against using HRT?

There are very few situations in which the potential risks of taking HRT are so high that it would be foolish to take it. Doctors use the term 'absolute contra-indications' for those, which are:

- pregnancy (!),
- active clotting problems in the veins (thrombosis),
- severe active liver disease,
- recurrence of cancer of the lining of the womb (endometrial cancer),
- recurrence of breast cancer.

In terms of numbers these 'absolute' categories count for only a small percentage of women who might be considering taking HRT, but for them it isn't a choice. A much bigger group of women are those for whom there are some increased risks, but which may not be so high that HRT is completely out of court. These are called 'relative contra-indications':

- abnormal vaginal bleeding – this must be properly investigated first,
- breast lump (prior to investigation),
- previous endometrial cancer,
- previous breast cancer,
- strong family history of breast cancer,
- previous vein thrombosis,
- family history of thrombosis,
- surgical operations (to reduce the risk of a vein thrombosis many surgeons advise women who are taking HRT to stop it four to six weeks prior to their operation if it is to be a major one involving a general anaesthetic).

It's impossible in a book of this nature to go further into the factors that are important in an individual woman, but when these 'relative' contra-indications are present then it needs a more compelling reason than usual to favour the use of HRT.

Although not in either of these lists, because it's not a 'medical' reason to do with safety, a woman's personal wishes are also of paramount importance. HRT is never compulsory, nor is it ever a life-saving or essential form of treatment. A woman should always have the last say about what treatment she will or won't have, and she is entitled to be fully informed in order to make that decision.

4. Which type of HRT?

If the decision is in favour of taking HRT then you will be well aware by now that the most important factor in choosing the type is whether a woman still has her uterus. If not, then she does not need progestogen and can choose from one of the various types of oestrogen-only tablets, patches, gels, nasal spray or local creams or vaginal rings.

Women with their uterus need combined HRT and those who are under 55 or are still having a period now and again should have the sequential type. Those who are a year or more past their last period or are about the age of 55 can go straight on to the continuous type of combined HRT. Women who start on sequential combined HRT should try to convert to one of the continuous types after a year or two.

As far as which brand to take is concerned this is often a matter of personal choice on behalf of the prescriber, rather than the patient. In the light of the HERS and WHI studies we can say that preparations that use conjugated oestrogens are going to become less popular, but that doesn't mean that women already taking them should stop doing so forthwith. All women taking HRT need to be aware of the risks and benefits, and the decision on which type of HRT to take needs to be discussed fully with the doctor. Most women receive supplies of HRT of about six months at a time from their GP, and the next routine check-up will usually be time enough to review the choice of prescription.

Unless a woman is at high risk of cardiovascular disease or vein thrombosis (in which case they should perhaps avoid HRT anyway) then any brand of appropriate HRT is fine for short-term use of up to a couple of years as far as we currently know. Once you start to extend the time or to use HRT in older women or those with extra risk factors, then the decision on what to use becomes more complex.

Often a trial and error approach is as good a way as any to finally choose the 'right' HRT as many of the deciding factors are not those of great import such as the long-term medical risks, but are of a more practical nature. You might find, for example, that you like the idea of patches but that your skin reacts to the adhesive, so you change brands and find another suits better. Or you move to tablets instead. Many HRT preparations have more than one available dose strength. Usually you'll start on the lowest and move to the higher dose if it doesn't control your symptoms adequately, and so on. There's both science and art in choosing HRT!

Key Points

- The first decision in menopause treatment is whether it is required at all. Sometimes the best you can do is to take it for a trial period to see if it helps.
- HRT, as opposed to other types of menopause treatment, needs to be considered in specific situations such as early menopause or when there is a high risk of osteoporosis.
- There are a small number of situations in which HRT should not be used at all, and a larger number in which the pros and cons need to be carefully balanced.
- The final judge on menopause treatment is the woman herself. HRT is never essential.

Chapter 9

The 'Male Menopause'

Does the 'male menopause' exist?

The heading of this paragraph is put as a question rather than a statement to reflect the controversy that surrounds the subject. Like a great many conditions that are revealed mainly, or only, by the symptoms that the patient experiences (rather than disturbances on a set of blood tests or body scans), many medical people are sceptical of the existence of the male menopause. Other conditions that get the same treatment include chronic fatigue (CFS/ME), fibromyalgia and irritable bowel syndrome.

People who have these problems, despite their often very significant symptoms, can find themselves not being taken seriously by those doctors and other health professionals who have an over-reliance on medical tests to determine if their patients are unwell. The short answer to the question though is definitely 'yes'. The difficulty, as with the female menopause, is in deciding when natural aging has merged into something more pervasive and which merits treatment.

Male aging

The testes are the main site of production of the male sex hormones, predominant among which is testosterone. Although men can retain the ability to produce active sperm in the testes throughout their lives the output of testosterone declines with age. Men undoubtedly experience symptoms caused by the drop in sex hormones but individuals are affected differently. Some men experience very few symptoms, whereas others are completely disabled by them. Although this fall in sex hormone production is a natural process and not a disease, this does not mean to say that the problem cannot and should not be diagnosed and treated when appropriate.

In women, as we've seen, the fall in oestrogen and progesterone production at the menopause can take some years to fully happen although in some women it can be more abrupt. The cessation of periods is an obvious outward sign that the menopause has occurred. In men the transition is usually slow, occurring over decades rather than years or months, and there is no obvious physical sign that is the male equivalent of periods stopping.

The mental and physical changes that can occur in men are much more subtle in onset and can easily be missed. As such, the term 'male menopause', or 'andropause', is probably not accurate. Instead, experts prefer to talk about 'partial androgen deficiency of the aging male' (PADAM).

Testosterone is not the only hormone that undergoes changes in production in an older man but the significance of the other hormones is even less clear.

Lack of research

A great deal of effort has gone into research on treatment for the menopause in women, but very little research has been undertaken into PADAM and the effects of treatment. A considerable body of literature exists about HRT in menopausal women, but hormone supplementation in aging men is highly controversial: a little evidence shows that such therapy is beneficial and equally little shows that it isn't! The quality of evidence in PADAM is therefore low, and many of the studies have been small, so the information has to be treated with some caution.

Androgens

Androgens are steroid hormones with specific effects on tissue growth (muscle, fat, skin, hair and others) and brain function. They have important roles in both men and women, but are produced in much larger quantities in men. In men, after puberty, the majority of androgens are produced by the testicles, mainly as testosterone. Other androgens – dehydroepiandrostenedione (DHEA), its sulphate (DHEAS), and dihydrotestosterone (DHT) – are produced in the adrenal glands (above the kidneys), skin and liver. Several man-made androgens are also available.

Androgen deficiency can occur in younger men, and even in children and adolescents, as a result of testicular damage, genetic disorders or metabolic disorders. It is very important that they receive expert assessment by an expert in hormone problems (endocrinologist) at an early stage and receive androgen replacement therapy. This is established medical practice and uncontroversial, unlike androgen supplementation therapy in PADAM.

The symptoms of androgen deficiency

The symptoms of PADAM are numerous and non-specific, so it is not an easy condition to diagnose. They include problems with:

Circulation and the nervous system:
- hot flushes
- sweating
- insomnia.

Mood and higher mental function:
- irritability and tiredness
- nervousness
- decreased sense of well-being
- lack of motivation
- low mental energy
- difficulty with short-term memory
- depression
- low self-esteem.

Masculinity and virility:
- decreased vigour and physical energy
- diminished muscle strength.

Sexuality:
- decreased interest in or desire for sex
- less sexual activity
- poor erections
- reduced quality of orgasm
- weakness of ejaculation
- reduced volume of ejaculated fluid.

Physical features include:
- diminished muscle mass
- loss of body hair
- abdominal obesity.

Several other effects on body chemistry and metabolism occur, such as:

- Changes in blood cholesterol pattern towards that which increases the risk of developing coronary artery disease.
- Increase in total body fat (because of a fall in the proportion of body weight that is muscle rather than through weight gain).
- Osteoporosis.

Many of these symptoms, signs and metabolic consequences can be corrected by androgen replacement therapy.

Diagnosing androgen deficiency (PADAM)

As with the female menopause, no definitive test for PADAM exists. Low blood levels of testosterone alone are insufficient to make the diagnosis. The combination of several different suggestive symptoms and physical signs, together with low blood levels of testosterone, should raise suspicion that PADAM is present.

TESTOSTERONE LEVELS
There are several reasons why diagnosing PADAM is not as easy as checking a man's testosterone level. Disagreement exists over what exactly should be measured in the blood to assess androgen deficiency and about what is the normal range of testosterone levels. The existing 'normal' range for total testosterone is based upon statistical analysis of pooled samples from all men, including those who might have PADAM.

So 'normal' testosterone levels are not necessarily the same as healthy levels.

Testosterone is released into the bloodstream in pulses, and levels vary through the day. In general, the testicles release more testosterone in the morning than later in the day. Blood samples should therefore be taken between 8 and 10am, and at least two separate, consistent results are needed to establish that there is a problem with testosterone levels.

About 60–70 per cent of the total testosterone is tightly bound to a protein, present in the blood, called sex hormone binding globulin (SHBG). This protein-binding is a common way in which hormones are transported in the bloodstream and it is effectively a circulating store of testosterone. The testosterone only becomes active when the link to SHBG is broken, and this is a process that occurs at a certain rate all the time. Older men produce relatively more SHBG, as do heavy drinkers and men with thyroid disorders, thus reducing the amount of 'free' testosterone.

Another 30–40 per cent of the total testosterone is more loosely bound to another protein, called albumen. Testosterone bound to albumen is also inactive, so free testosterone probably accounts for only 1–2 per cent of the total. Measurement of total testosterone is therefore a poor measure of active testosterone. Free testosterone levels are expensive to measure and are not widely available.

Free Androgen Index (FAI = total testosterone/SHBG ×100) is an alternative measure of androgen state that is not as reliable as free testosterone, but is better than relying solely on total testosterone. All this is confusing for doctors, too!

Treatment

Many doctors do not believe that PADAM exists and will not offer treatment. Others are 'believers' and see it everywhere. At present, a practical approach is probably the most helpful. If multiple symptoms of PADAM are present and the free androgen index (FAI) is below normal or in the lower part of the normal range, a 'therapeutic trial' of testosterone supplement therapy for up to three months can be worthwhile. If there has been no improvement in symptoms, despite a rise in FAI after three months of therapy, then continuation of treatment is probably not worthwhile. If there is an improvement in symptoms, persevering with treatment is worthwhile for as long as the improvement is maintained. A very high placebo response to treatment probably occurs, so it is important to check that the improvement is maintained over time.

Men receiving testosterone supplements should have regular medical checks every three months for the first year of treatment, which must include a rectal examination of the prostate gland (which sits beneath the bladder producing fluids that nourish and protect sperm) and blood tests. After that period, at least yearly checks are necessary.

FORMS OF TREATMENT

Testosterone preparations are available as capsules, injections, patches and implants. Capsules do not always provide steady blood levels. Patches are probably the easiest form of testosterone to take, although they are fairly expensive. All these preparations can be prescribed on the NHS, although a GP would be unlikely to agree to prescribe these medications for PADAM without a specialist's advice.

SIDE EFFECTS

Headache, weight gain, acne, increased aggression and male-pattern baldness have all been reported with testosterone treatment, but are uncommon if free testosterone levels are maintained within the normal range.

Considerable controversy exists over the effect of testosterone upon the prostate gland. Men with abnormally low levels of testosterone have small prostate glands. Replacement therapy causes the prostate to grow to about the average size predicted for their age. Current evidence indicates that testosterone does not cause abnormal prostate enlargement (benign prostatic hypertrophy). Testosterone should not be given to men who have symptoms of restricted urine flow (urinary outflow obstruction) due to prostate enlargement.

Testosterone supplements are not thought to cause prostate cancer. However, the hormone does help existing prostate cancers grow and must not be given to men with prostate cancer. If a man lives long enough, he will probably develop prostate cancer (up to 80 per cent of 80-year-old men are found to have prostate cancer at post-mortem examination) so whether testosterone supplements will affect mortality in older men is unknown.

Cholesterol levels and production of red blood cells are affected by testosterone, and must be closely monitored, particularly during the first year of treatment.

Osteoporosis in men

Like oestrogen in women testosterone has a protective effect on bone and osteoporosis in men was mentioned briefly at the end of chapter 7.

Awareness of osteoporosis in men is still rather low, including among health professionals. Suspicion should be raised though in a man who has had a fracture at a relatively young age, for example, or after relatively little trauma, or who shows signs of height loss or whose spine X-rays are suggestive of some bone loss. Men can also benefit from all of the general and more specific treatments, other than HRT, that apply to women. The exact role of testosterone treatment in male osteoporosis is uncertain because insufficient research has been done into the condition. Unless testosterone levels are very low then there are the difficulties referred to above in establishing whether androgen deficiency does or does not exist.

Osteoporosis treatment in men is therefore presently along the lines of encouraging exercise and an adequate diet, using supplements if necessary. Bisphosphonate drugs can be used when more active treatment is required.

Key Points

- Androgen deficiency in older men (PADAM) is controversial, but it is increasingly accepted as a real condition.
- Diagnosis is based on the pattern of symptoms allied to careful interpretation of blood results.
- The long-term benefit of testosterone supplements in older men with symptoms of PADAM is unclear.
- Testosterone treatment is probably worth trying in men with disabling symptoms, provided that they are properly counselled and receive adequate follow-up.
- Osteoporosis in men is real, and under-diagnosed.
- More research is needed to clarify this controversial area.

Chapter 10

Other Issues at the Menopause

Contraception in older women

Although a woman's peak fertility begins to decline in her 30s this is now the commonest decade in which women give birth in the UK. Fertility is arbitrarily presumed to have disappeared by two years after the last period for women under 50 years old, and one year in women 50 or older. Many women going through the climacteric therefore need to consider what to do about contraception.

TYPES OF HORMONAL CONTRACEPTION

Contraceptive hormones are of two main types. The 'combined oral contraceptive' is what most people mean by 'The Pill', and like combined HRT it contains both oestrogen and progestogen. The relatively high levels of oestrogen and progestogen that result from taking the Pill prevent the brain and pituitary gland from releasing the hormones that in turn cause the development and release of eggs from a woman's ovaries, hence the contraceptive effect. In a way, the Pill fools the brain into thinking that the woman is pregnant, and thus further pregnancy is prevented.

The 'mini-pill' contains only progestogen and works by making fertilisation of the egg by sperm more difficult. It also makes the environment within the uterus hostile to a fertilised egg, thus preventing it from implanting. On progestogen-only contraception eggs may still be released but this happens erratically.

Long-acting progestogen-only contraceptives include the three-monthly contraceptive injection (Depo-Provera®) and implants such as Implanon®, which lasts up to three years and is inserted under the skin of the upper arm. The latter can be removed if side effects develop whereas once the injection has been given, it's there until it wears off.

CONTRACEPTION AND HRT

The levels of hormone used in contraceptive pills and injections are several times more powerful than those in HRT. HRT has no contraceptive powers. Conversely a woman taking the oral contraceptive will have more than enough circulating oestrogen to prevent her from experiencing any menopausal symptoms.

Even if her Pill is masking the symptoms, a woman's ovaries are still getting older, slowly declining in function and eventually will cease to have any capacity to generate more eggs should the contraception be stopped.

It would be very handy indeed if we had a test to say when it was safe to stop taking any contraception, but for the same reasons as there is no lab test for the menopause, we don't have one that guarantees a woman's fertility, or lack of it. The one or two years' rule mentioned at the start of this chapter has been found by experience to be reliable, but it is not guaranteed.

CONTRACEPTIVE CHOICES IN OLDER WOMEN

There are risks attached to hormonal contraception containing oestrogen, and they are similar to those we've already covered in connection with HRT. The main one is the increased tendency to develop clots in the veins and this risk increases in older women. Combined oral contraception (the Pill) can be continued up to the age of around 50 years but only in women who do not smoke and who have no other risk factors such as obesity or high blood pressure. Women who smoke should be advised to stop the combined pill at the age of 35 years. However, the progestogen-containing methods of hormonal contraception can be easily continued until age 50 by most women as they are very safe and have very few risks attached to taking them.

There are many potential solutions to the contraception issue, which is a subject that could easily fill a book on its own. The main options for a peri-menopausal woman are:

- **Sterilisation** of either the male or female partner. Male sterilisation by vasectomy is a simple and quick procedure that can be done under local anaesthetic. Female sterilisation is now routinely done by 'keyhole surgery' but still involves a general anaesthetic. Sterilisation immediately removes the need for a woman to take any more hormones for contraception. But it has significant risks at a time when a woman's fertility is already much reduced.
- **Intra-uterine device**. The IUD is an effective form of contraception that can be particularly appropriate to a peri-menopausal woman. It avoids the need for hormonal contraception and can usually be left in place for five years before needing replacement. Because fertility declines with age, for most women an IUD put in after their fortieth birthday will last them well into the post-

menopausal part of their lives without needing to be changed, when they can forget about contraception. Mirena® can kill three birds with one stone by providing a low dose of progestogen inside the uterus (which can control erratic vaginal bleeding *and* provide adequate protection of the uterus to allow the use of oestrogen-only HRT), in addition to being an even more effective contraceptive than the standard IUD.

- **Barrier methods** of contraception such as condoms, diaphragms and caps can be useful options for an older woman, even if she's not previously used them. If well used these are very close to as good as hormonal contraception in effectiveness but if one also takes into account that an older woman's level of fertility is reduced (even if not yet zero) then this may make barrier methods more effective compared to younger women. Practical problems such as a lack of lubrication of the vagina may make them more difficult to use but these can be overcome with suitable lubricant gels.
- **'Natural' family planning** using the rhythm method, temperature charts and so on are not the best methods of contraception at the best of times but near the menopause, when a woman's cycle is even less predictable, they are much less reliable and can't be recommended.

The correct choice of contraception, at any age, is always an individual one based on a woman's particular circumstances and desires. This is no less the case at the end of a woman's reproductive years.

Future trends in menopause treatment

As we've clearly seen, HRT is not a panacea for the menopause. Correctly used it can confer benefits but it has its downsides. Much of the current research interest in the development of treatments for the menopause is focussed on trying to develop medicines that provide the benefits without the disadvantages. SERMs (selective estrogen receptor modulators) are currently the drugs that hold out the most promise. We know that there are different types of oestrogen 'receptor' in different tissues, so the search is on for SERMs that help flushes and sweats and protect bones but which do not stimulate breast and endometrial tissue or activate the tendency for clots to form in veins. We should hopefully see positive results from such research in the next few years.

General health

We've mentioned more than once already that there is a tendency to think of the menopause as an illness or a health hazard, which is the wrong way to look at it. It's a phase of life and like all such things we have to live with it. The hand of woman (or man) has little influence on the processes of nature, and you'll be aware now if you weren't before that the menopause is a changing scene in the world of medicine. There are many unanswered questions, and many of the problems that we thought we knew some of the answers to have turned out not to be so clear-cut.

The big health issues that face older women in the UK today are mainly to do with cardiovascular diseases, being overweight, developing diabetes and having poor mental health. It's the same list for men. We know of the extra things to do with these problems that need attention across the population: the low level of exercise that most of us take; our excessive intake of high calorie foods, salt and alcohol; the presence of high blood pressure and cholesterol levels. These are actually bigger threats than cancer to the majority of people, and all of them can be heavily influenced to the better by actions that we can take ourselves.

It's perhaps taking it a bit far to say that with the right attitude the menopause can be made into a joyous part of your life. However, the same actions that make life better generally will make the menopause better too.

Appendix A

References

General

- Dell, D. L., and Stewart, D. E., 'Menopause and mood' (Postgraduate medicine online, September 2000); http://www.postgradmed.com/issues/2000/09_00/dell.htm

NHS Cancer screening services information

- Breast: http://www.cancerscreening.nhs.uk/breastscreen/index.html
- Cervix: http://www.cancerscreening.nhs.uk/cervical/index.html

Hormone replacement therapy

- Stevenson, J. C., and Whitehead, M. I., 'Editorial' (concerning women's health initiative trial) (British Medical Journal, 2002; 325: 113–14); http://bmj.com/cgi/content/full/325/7356/113
- Rymer, J., et al., 'Making decisions about hormone replacement therapy' (British Medical Journal, 2003; 326: 322–26); http://bmj.com/cgi/content/full/326/7384/322
- Writing group for the WHI study, 'Risks and benefits of estrogen plus progestin in healthy postmenopausal women: principal results from the women's health initiative randomised controlled trial' (Journal of the American Medical Association, 2002; 288: 321–33); http://jama.ama-assn.org/cgi/content/abstract/288/3/321
- Grady, D., et al., 'Cardiovascular disease outcomes during 6.8 years of hormone therapy: heart and estrogen/progestin replacement study (HERS II)' (Journal of the American Medical Association, 2002; 288: 49–57); http://jama.ama-assn.org/cgi/content/abstract/288/1/49
- Hulley, S., et al., 'Noncardiovascular disease outcomes during 6.8 years of hormone therapy: heart and estrogen/progestin replacement study (HERS II)' (Journal of the American Medical Association, 2002; 288: 58–66); http://jama.ama-assn.org/cgi/content/abstract/288/1/58
- Shumaker, S. A., et al., 'Estrogen plus progestin and the incidence of dementia and mild cognitive impairment in postmenopausal women: the women's health initiative memory study' (Journal of the American Medical Association, 2003; 289(20): 2651–62); http://jama.ama-assn.org/cgi/content/abstract/289/20/2651
- Wassertheil-Smoller, S., et al., 'Effect of estrogen plus progestin on stroke in postmenopausal women: the women's health initiative' (Journal of the American Medical Association, 2003; 289(20): 2673–84); http://jama.ama-assn.org/cgi/content/abstract/289/20/2673

Complementary treatments

- Davis, S. R., 'Phytoestrogen therapy for menopausal symptoms?' (British Medical Journal, 2001; 323: 354–55); http://bmj.com/cgi/content/full/323/7309/354
- Kass-Annese, B., 'Alternative therapies for menopause' (Clinical Obstetrics and Gynecology, 2000; 43(1): 162–83).

Breast disease

- Dixon, J. M., 'Hormone replacement therapy and the breast' (British Medical Journal, 2001; 323: 1381–82); http://bmj.com/cgi/content/full/323/7326/1381

Osteoporosis

- Cummings, S. R., and Melton, L. J., 'Epidemiology and outcomes of osteoporotic fractures' (Lancet, 2002; 18: 1714).
- Primary Care Strategy for Osteoporosis and Falls (National Osteoporosis Society); http://www.nos.org.uk/PDF/PCGDoc2002.pdf
- Scottish Intercollegiate Guidelines Network (SIGN) Guideline 71: 'Management of Osteoporosis' (June 2003); http://www.sign.ac.uk/pdf/sign71.pdf

'Male menopause'

- Gould, D. C., et al., 'The male menopause – does it exist?' (British Medical Journal, 2000; 320: 858–61); http://bmj.com/cgi/content/full/320/7238/858

Appendix B

Drugs Used for the Menopause

The following information contains selected details of some of the medications used in treating the menopause. Full details are included in the manufacturers' data sheets and can also be viewed within the medicines section of the NetDoctor web site: http://www.netdoctor.co.uk/medicines/

The information is accurate at the time of writing but new information on medicines appears regularly. A health professional should always be consulted concerning the prescription and use of medicines.

Medicines and their possible side effects can affect individual people in different ways. The following lists some of the side effects that are known to be associated with these medicines. Side effects other than those listed may exist.

There are many available brands of hormone replacement therapy, containing oestrogen alone or oestrogen combined with a progestogen.

The potential side effects of all these types of HRT are very similar. The following information is generally applicable to all types.

Combined HRT

Combined HRT contains forms of the naturally occurring female sex hormones, oestrogen and progesterone.

In women with an intact womb, oestrogen stimulates the growth of the womb lining (endometrium). This can lead to endometrial cancer if the growth is unopposed. For this reason it is essential that women with an intact womb be given a progesterone to oppose oestrogen's effect on the womb lining. If a woman has had her womb surgically removed (a hysterectomy), endometrial cancer is not a risk and progesterone is not necessary as part of HRT. As this medicine contains both an oestrogen and a progesterone it is suitable for women who have not had a hysterectomy.

There are two main types of HRT. One type gives a continuous daily dose of both hormones, which normally results in the stopping of menstrual periods. This type, called continuous HRT, is recommended for women who are at least 12 months after their last natural menstrual bleed.

The other type of HRT uses the concept of 'cycle therapy'. In cycle (also called 'sequential') therapy the progesterone component is added for 10–14 days at the end of the cycle. This mimics the fluctuating levels of oestrogen and progesterone that occur in the natural menstrual cycle and results in the womb lining being shed as a menstrual period at the end of each month. Sequential combined HRT is usually used in women who have not yet ceased menstruation but who are otherwise deemed to need HRT.

MAIN SIDE EFFECTS

Women taking HRT appear to have a small increase in the risk of being diagnosed with breast cancer, compared with women who do not take HRT. However, this risk must be weighed against the benefits of taking HRT, such as prevention of osteoporosis. Women on HRT are advised to have regular breast examinations and mammograms, and to practise breast self-examination.

Women taking HRT have a slight increase in the risk of abnormal blood clot formation (deep vein thrombosis and pulmonary embolism) compared with women not taking HRT. The Committee for the Safety of Medicines believes that the overall benefits of HRT outweigh the risks involved, but that those with a personal or family history of thrombosis or other risk factors (e.g. severe varicose veins, obesity, recent surgery, immobility) should carefully discuss this with their doctor.

Stop taking this medicine and inform your doctor immediately if you experience any of the following whilst taking this medicine: stabbing pains or swelling in the legs, pain on breathing or coughing, shortness of breath, worsening of epilepsy, migraine or severe headaches, visual disturbances, severe abdominal complaints, increased blood pressure, itching of the whole body or yellowing of the skin and eyes (jaundice).

Irregular breakthrough bleeding may occur in the first few months of treatment with this medicine, usually followed by your periods stopping completely. If you experience prolonged bleeding, or start to bleed again after a long bleed-free time, or after stopping treatment consult your doctor.

OTHER POSSIBLE SIDE EFFECTS

- headache
- dizziness or loss of balance
- fatigue

- awareness of the heartbeat (palpitations)
- excessive fluid retention in the body tissues, resulting in swelling (oedema)
- nosebleeds
- vaginal discharge
- hair loss
- high blood pressure
- skin reactions such as rash and itch
- depressed mood
- changes in sex drive
- gut disturbances such as heartburn, nausea, vomiting, bloating, wind and stomach pain
- build-up of bile (biliary stasis)
- breast tenderness/swelling/pain

USE WITH CAUTION IN:
- asthma
- benign breast lumps (fibrocystic breast disease) or a history of this
- impaired heart or kidney function
- diabetes
- disorder causing deafness in adult life (otosclerosis)
- epilepsy
- fibroids of the uterus
- gallstones
- high blood pressure
- high levels of calcium in the blood
- lifelong inherited blood diseases (porphyrias)
- systemic lupus erythematosus
- disorders of bile excretion such as Dubin-Johnson syndrome and Rotor syndrome
- migraine
- multiple sclerosis

- a history of recurrent blood clots in the veins (venous thrombo-embolism) who are taking anticoagulant medicines
- diseases where there is a tendency for the blood to clot in the veins (thrombophilic disease) who are taking anticoagulant medicines
- personal or family history of blood clots in the veins (venous thromboembolism)
- severe obesity

NOT TO BE USED IN:
- history of breast cancer
- known or suspected breast cancer
- known or suspected cancer responsive to female hormones (oestrogen dependent neoplasia) e.g. endometrial cancer
- people who have had a deep vein thrombosis in the last 2 years
- people who have had a pulmonary embolism in the last 2 years
- people with a history of recurrent blood clots in the veins (venous thromboembolism) who are not taking anticoagulant medicines
- people with diseases that cause a tendency for the blood to clot in the veins (thrombophilic disease) who are not taking anticoagulant medicines
- pre-menopausal women
- pregnancy or suspected pregnancy
- severe heart disease
- severe kidney disease
- severe liver disease
- vaginal bleeding of unknown cause

INTERACTIONS WITH OTHER MEDICINES
The blood levels and effects of this medicine may be reduced when it is taken with the following:

- rifamycins such as rifabutin and rifampicin
- antiepileptic medicines such as carbamazepine, phenytoin, pheno-barbital and primidone
- barbiturates such as amobarbital (amylobarbitone)
- the herbal remedy St John's wort

This may result in recurrence of symptoms. Tell your doctor if you are taking any other medicines before starting HRT. This medicine may increase the blood levels of ciclosporin or ropinirole if either of these medicines are taken at the same time.

Selective estrogen receptor modulator (SERM) – Raloxifene (Evista®)

HOW DOES IT WORK?

Raloxifene is a selective estrogen receptor modulator (SERM). It has actions similar to those of oestrogens on bone tissue, but not on uterine or breast tissues.

At the menopause blood levels of oestrogen (the main female sex hormone) decrease, which leads to a loss of bone density. Bone loss is particularly rapid for the first ten years after the menopause. This may lead to the development of osteoporosis – a condition in which the bones are brittle and break more easily.

Raloxifene binds to oestrogen receptors and stimulates their action in bone and the cardiovascular system. This leads to an eventual increase in the density of bone.

Raloxifene is used to treat post-menopausal osteoporosis. It is not useful in the treatment of menopausal symptoms such as hot flushes.

USE WITH CAUTION IN:

- immobility
- those with risk factors for developing blood clots, such as obesity, immobility, varicose veins or a history of blood clot disorders

NOT TO BE USED IN:

- blood clot in the blood vessels (acute thromboembolism)
- breast cancer
- decreased liver function
- endometrial cancer
- failure of normal bile flow to the intestine (cholestasis)
- known sensitivity or allergy to any ingredient
- severe kidney disease
- vaginal bleeding of unknown cause
- women of child-bearing age

MAIN POTENTIAL SIDE EFFECTS

- swelling of the legs and ankles due to excess fluid retention (peripheral oedema)
- leg cramps
- hot flushes
- blood clot in the veins
- inflammation of the vein wall (thrombophlebitis)

INTERACTION WITH OTHER MEDICINES

The absorption of raloxifene is reduced by cholestyramine and it is recommended that they are not used together. When used together with warfarin or nicoumalone, raloxifene may reduce the blood thinning effects of these medicines.

Tibolone (Livial®)

Tibolone is a synthetic steroid that mimics the activity of oestrogen and progesterone (female sex hormones) in the body.

WHAT IS IT USED FOR?
- hot flushes and sweating caused by hormonal disturbances during the menopause
- to help prevent the development of osteoporosis

MAIN POTENTIAL SIDE EFFECTS
- rash
- depression
- disturbances of the gut such as diarrhoea, constipation, nausea, vomiting or abdominal pain
- visual disturbances
- pain in the muscles (myalgia)
- weight changes
- headache
- swelling of the legs and ankles due to excess fluid retention (peripheral oedema)
- dizziness
- growth of facial hair

Bisphosphonate – Alendronate (Fosamax®)

HOW DOES IT WORK?
This medicine contains the active ingredient alendronate sodium, which is a type of medicine called a bisphosphonate. These agents are used in a variety of metabolic bone disorders. Bone cells continuously deposit and remove calcium and phosphorus, stored in a protein network that makes up the structure of bone. Biphosphonates work by

binding very tightly to bone crystals, preventing the removal of calcium. This decreases breakdown and turnover of bone in the body and the increased calcium content leads to stronger bones.

In osteoporosis, bone turnover is increased, causing the bones to become weak and prone to breaking. This medicine slows down the process of bone breakdown, so keeping bones stronger and helping to prevent fractures. It is used to treat osteoporosis and prevent fractures in people with the disease, and also to prevent bone loss in people at risk of developing osteoporosis.

It is important that the dosing instructions for this medicine are followed completely. This is because the medicine can cause irritation and ulceration of the gullet (oesophagus). Following the instructions correctly minimises this risk. The tablets must be swallowed whole with a glass of plain water (at least 200ml, not mineral water), and not sucked or chewed. You should sit or stand for at least 30 minutes after taking the tablet to aid its movement into the stomach. For this reason don't take the tablet before getting up in the morning or less than 30 minutes before going to bed at night.

MAIN POTENTIAL SIDE EFFECTS
- headache
- rash
- flatulence
- other disturbances of the gut such as heartburn, diarrhoea, constipation, nausea, vomiting or abdominal pain
- low blood calcium level (hypocalcaemia)
- pain in muscles or bones (musculoskeletal pain)
- flushing of the skin
- inflammation of the food pipe (oesophagitis)
- abnormal reaction of the skin to light, usually a rash (photosensitivity)
- inflammation of the front parts of the eye (uveitis)

INTERACTIONS WITH OTHER MEDICINES

Calcium supplements, antacids and possibly some other medicines taken by mouth may interfere with the absorption of this medicine from the gut. For this reason you should wait at least 30 minutes after taking alendronate, before taking any other medicines by mouth.

Clonidine (Dixarit®)

HOW DOES IT WORK?

Clonidine is thought to reduce the responsiveness of small blood vessels to stimuli that would normally make them contract (narrow) or dilate (widen). This prevents the changes in the blood vessels of the brain that are associated with migraine, and thus prevents attacks. It also prevents the dilatation of blood vessels and subsequent increased blood flow to the skin, which causes hot flushes in post-menopausal women. It may take two to four weeks before this medicine is fully effective. Clonidine is used in higher doses to treat high blood pressure.

MAIN POTENTIAL SIDE EFFECTS

- headache
- constipation
- dry mouth
- drowsiness
- confusion
- false perceptions of things that are not really there (hallucinations)
- pins and needles (paraesthesia)
- dizziness
- nausea and vomiting
- drop in blood pressure occurring when going from lying down to sitting or standing, which can cause light-headedness
- hair loss (alopecia)
- dry eyes (which can affect contact lens wearers)

- decreased sex drive
- depressed mood

POSSIBLE INTERACTIONS WITH OTHER MEDICINES

Tricyclic antidepressants such as amitriptyline may reduce the effectiveness of clonidine.

When taken together with a beta-blocker such as atenolol, there is a risk of a rebound increase in blood pressure if the patient stops taking clonidine. To prevent this, the beta-blocker should be stopped several days before slowly stopping the clonidine.

When taken together with a beta-blocker or cardiac glycoside (e.g. digoxin) there may be a slowing of the heart rate or an abnormal heart rhythm.

This medicine may increase the effects of medicines that lower blood pressure either as their main action, or as a side effect. This can result in dizziness or light-headedness.

Appendix C

Useful Contacts

The Amarant Trust

The Menopause Amarant Trust is a charity that aims to help women deal with problems they might experience while going through the menopause. The aims are met by a nurse-staffed telephone helpline, a clinic, leaflets and booklets and medical staff study days.

Tel: 01293 413000
www.amarantmenopausetrust.org.uk

The Daisy Network

The Daisy Network (previously known as the Daisy Chain) is a registered charity and support group for women suffering premature menopause.

Email: membership&media@daisynetwork.org.uk
www.daisynetwork.org.uk

National Osteoporosis Society

A national charity dedicated to improving the diagnosis, prevention and treatment of osteoporosis.

Tel: 01761 471771 (general enquiries)
Helpline: 01761 472721
www.nos.org.uk

Women's Health Concern

A charitable organisation working to support women dealing with the menopause and other gynaecological conditions.

Helpline: 01628 488065
www.womens-health-concern.org

Institute for Complementary Medicine

A registered charity that provides the public with information on Complementary Medicine. It administers the British Register of Complementary Practitioners (BRCP), which is a register of professional, competent practitioners.

Tel: 020 7237 5165
www.icmedicine.co.uk

National Institute of Medical Herbalists

The UK's leading professional association of practitioners of herbal medicine. It administers a register of trained herbalists.

Tel: 01392 426022
www.nimh.org.uk

British Homeopathic Association

A charity that promotes education and research into homeopathy. Its website includes a directory of health professionals trained in homeopathy.

Tel: 0870 444 3950
www.trusthomeopathy.org